Yoga

The founder of the AtréYoga Studio in New Delhi, **Zubin Atré** has more than 9,000 hours of experience teaching yoga. He has designed sports yoga programmes for ace athletes, stress and energy management courses for multinationals and transformational programmes for couples and individuals.

Dipping into his knowledge of the human anatomy, yoga and psychology, Zubin has developed a unique style of teaching. This comprises a series of meticulously crafted asanas, all of which convey his commitment to detail, to an interactive learning experience and to making the wisdom of yoga relevant to real-life situations.

Zubin writes regularly for and has been featured in major publications, newspapers and magazines, besides appearing in television shows in India and abroad. He holds a degree in business, and when not teaching yoga, likes to travel, learn languages, write and go exploring by motorbike (this, he refers to as a form of meditation).

Zubin divides his time between Asia and Europe, conducting workshops and retreats. You can learn more about him and his programmes at www.zubinatre.com and www. atreyogastudio.com and follow him on Twitter @zubinatre.

Models: Zubin Atré is the male model. Sara Zennaro Atré, the female model, is a certified yoga teacher. She has been practising yoga since her childhood. She has carried her passion for yoga with her across several countries in Latin America, the Middle East and Asia, where she has lived and worked as an international civil servant.

It Takes Two To Yoga

Asanas for Couples & Partners

Zubin Atré

RUPA

Published by
Rupa Publications India Pvt. Ltd 2016
7/16, Ansari Road, Daryaganj
New Delhi 110002

Sales Centres:

Allahabad Bengaluru Chennai
Hyderabad Jaipur Kathmandu
Kolkata Mumbai

ISBN: 978-81-291-3967-2

First impression 2016

10 9 8 7 6 5 4 3 2 1

The moral right of the author has been asserted.

Printed by Parksons Graphics Pvt. Ltd, Mumbai

To my brother Ashish Atré
whose trust in me never fails to surprise me

CONTENTS

A NOTE FROM THE AUTHOR

Everyone can practise partner yoga, from parents and children, to husbands and wives, and colleagues. The asanas technically remain the same no matter what the nature of the collaboration is. However, the form of non-verbal communication, the energy, the emotions and, by consequence, the benefits associated with the asanas, will vary based on one's association with one's companion.

No prior yogic experience is required to practise partner yoga. However, be gentle with your body if you are a beginner. Remember that you are not in competition with anyone else. Also, always maintain a positive outlook. This is particularly important in the context of partner yoga since it is fun! You'll find yourself laughing with your yoga-buddy about the postures you are attempting. You might lose your balance, and may have to start from scratch, but finally, when you secure a good grip of your partner's ankles, wrists or arms, you will not only enjoy completing the asana, but also have memories that are truly amusing.

In addition, while attempting to get comfortable in a posture, remember the no-one-asana-fits-all rule. Each individual has a specific body structure, a different level of flexibility and strength. So, instead of forcing the body into the perfect pose, the serious yoga practitioner adapts an asana to suit her/his body type, flexibility or strength and medical history. In other words, the asana should fit the yogi and not the other way around.

Finally, always consult a physician to evaluate your medical condition before attempting any kind of yoga, and follow the medical advice you are given.

INTRODUCTION

IT'S ALL ABOUT TOUCH:
AN INITIATION INTO PARTNER YOGA

On the ceiling of the Sistine Chapel in Vatican City, we can see a beautiful fresco—Michelangelo's 'Creation of Adam'—with God stretching out his finger to grant Adam the spark of life. This is how the story begins—not just of Adam, but of all mankind. With touch. To quote Michelangelo: 'To touch can be to give life'.

Therefore, when two people meld—when they adopt partner yoga, instead of individual yoga—the impact and the experience of their practice deepens on account of touch.

To understand the features and benefits of partner yoga, we have to start from the most basic unit—just as we would start with the foundation if we had to build a house. In this case, we must begin with the full appreciation of a term—yoga. Born in India thousands of years ago, yoga means 'union' and is derived from the 'yoking together' of the mind and the body. Its practice helps one transcend the physical and mental planes to establish a spiritual union with the divine (usually experienced while in a deep state of meditation).

The intent guiding yoga, therefore, goes beyond acquiring a physically fit, astonishingly flexible body. But the practice of yoga must start at the physical level with an asana or posture. Yogic asanas are vital for the practitioner to develop both the physical strength to hold a stable and comfortable meditative position, and the mental strength and focus to calm the restless mind.

THE IMPORTANCE OF TOUCH

Interestingly enough, touch is the first of the five senses that human beings develop when they are still in their mother's womb—as early as in the eighth week after conception. The first part of a baby's body to experience any kind of sensitivity is the cheek. This sensation quickly extends to the palms at eleven weeks, and the soles of the feet at twelve weeks. In the womb, the baby experiments with this newfound sense of touch by stroking her or his face or sucking on a thumb, as well as feeling other body parts and seeing how they move. In the last trimester of pregnancy, when space becomes an issue, the baby's body presses against the womb-wall. Gentle patting and stroking alerts the baby to the mother's touch, and the baby may respond by calming down or kicking and nudging.

After birth, during the first few months of life, babies rely on grown-ups for tactile stimulation and comfort. They don't move much initially, but by the fourth month, they are able to reach out and touch whatever is nearby, such as blankets, toys and a parent's face. At about eight months, babies can touch and identify familiar objects without seeing them. In other words, their tactile sense actually helps them understand what the object is. The skin becomes the first point of physical contact with the outside world.

As babies grow, it is through such physical contact that they are able to 'feel' the world and make sense of their physical beings. It is through tactile sensation that they are able to find pleasure in holding a warm blanket on a cold winter morning, or find joy in a dog rubbing against their feet.

THE PHYSIOLOGY OF TOUCH

The skin is composed of several layers. At the very top is the epidermis, which is the layer we can see. Made primarily of dead skin cells, the epidermis is waterproof and serves as a protective wrap for the underlying skin layers and the rest of the body. It contains melanin, which acts as a shield against the sun's harmful rays and also gives the skin its colour. Besides, the epidermis contains very sensitive cells called touch receptors that give the brain information about the surrounding environment.

Below the epidermis is the dermis, which contains hair follicles, sweat glands, oil glands, blood vessels, nerve endings and a variety of touch receptors. Its primary function is to sustain and support the epidermis by diffusing nutrients to it and replacing the skin cells that are shed from the upper layer of the epidermis.

Then there is the hypodermis, composed of elastin, fat and connective tissue. The layer of fat acts as an insulator and helps regulate body temperature, besides serving as a cushion to protect underlying tissue from damage.

So, how do we feel things? Simply put, our sense of touch is controlled by a vast network of nerve endings and touch receptors in the skin known as the somato-sensory system. This system is responsible for all the sensations we feel—cold, hot, smooth, rough, ticklish, itchy, painful. Once a touch sensation is felt on the skin's somato-sensory network, the nervous system helps transmit signals to the brain. The brain then processes this information and communicates it back to the body.

Touch also has memory, known as 'haptic memory'. The human brain can remember several touch sensations and can also consciously retrieve a *specific* one from the past. A new touch sensation registered in one's memory does not erase recollections of a previous touch.

Proprioception

A key element related to touch, that is especially important for yoga practice, is proprioception. Have you ever wondered how you are able to press the accelerator while driving your car, without actually looking for it each time? This ability of the central nervous system to communicate with and coordinate various parts of the body—sometimes colloquially referred to as the 'sixth sense'—is, known as proprioception.

The word proprioception comes from a combination of the Latin word 'proprius', meaning 'one's own' and 'perception'. It is, therefore, a perception of self or, more specifically, a perception of where your body is and what it is doing. While the sense of touch is essentially external, as it collects information from the outside world, proprioception collects information from the body itself.

Proprioception is part of your everyday life. Even apparently simple actions like holding a pen, a cup or your partner's hand requires proprioception, in addition, of course, to the sensation of touch. Accordingly, as you will observe later on, proprioception is what will allow you to get into a yogic asana with your companion and maintain your posture—even if your eyes are closed, or your back is turned to your partner or you're hanging in an inverted position!

Kinaesthetic Awareness

Another important term that is crucial to understand the subtleties surrounding asanas is kinaesthetic awareness. Emerging from the Greek word 'kinesis', or 'motion' and the Latin word 'sentire', or 'to feel', kinaesthetic awareness is the body's ability to root itself in time and space and remain coordinated while engaging the outside world. By providing information through receptors about muscles, tendons, joints and other body parts, kinaesthetic awareness helps control and synchronize multiple activities—for example, jogging while talking. Similarly, when people in a group walk together, it is largely kinaesthetic awareness that allows them to move in harmony without bumping into one another. Consequently, while proprioception is an inner sense (linked to the central nervous system), kinaesthetic awareness is an external sense, and both work together and affect each other.

Every human being possesses kinaesthetic awareness in varying degrees. Without it you would have to use your eyes before you moved. For instance, to shift your leg, you do not need to look at it; without your kinaesthetic sense, however, you'd have to stare at your leg before moving it since you'd find it impossible to sense its position, or guess how much effort would have to be exerted to lift it.

With yogic practice, it is your kinaesthetic sense that allows you to maintain your balance in an asana, as it helps determine your orientation. In the case of partner yoga, kinaesthetic awareness helps you place your body in space and time in relation to your companion's position.

THE PSYCHOLOGY OF TOUCH

You've probably noticed how a hug from a loved one makes you feel valued and special (and hey, it can lower your blood pressure, too!), or how a firm handshake with a friend can build a connection. The ways in which human beings perceive a hug or a handshake, and the ways in which touch receptors receive the pressure of the arms or of the hand, are rooted in the brain. There are several kinds of touch:

▶ Intimate touch: If a person you care for hugs you, you will most likely experience a feeling of warmth and comfort. This is because your pressure sensors—which respond to all touch, whether it is a handshake, a hug or a kiss—send a message to your brain which helps it decode the quality of the embrace; your brain, in case the touch is intimate, will interpret the nature of the hug as pleasant, and this brings you joy.

▶ Healing or therapeutic touch: This type of touch is often associated with a massage or acupuncture. The pressure, in this case, can be gentle (for instance, a massage meant to soothe sore muscles). It can also be hard and delve deep (for instance, when a masseur works on the knots on the back muscles as part of a deep tissue massage). Despite differences in the severity of pressure, when you receive this kind of touch you are likely to be aware that the outcome will be healing, so your body allows you to relax.

▶ Exploratory or inquisitive touch: When you test foods or fabrics or try to identify objects by surveying their textures, you are learning about the world through the sense of touch. When it concerns objects which you deal with frequently in your daily life, it is possible to rely solely on the sense of touch to identify them. This is why it's easy for you to reach into your bag and find a bunch of keys without looking at them directly. Your brain recognizes the cold feeling of metal and the hard but smooth texture of your plastic key chain, or the rough finish of a jute bag.

▶ Aggressive or painful touch: You have likely experienced a kind of touch that can be equated with pain; this happens if the pressure applied is far too intense or the intent is wrong and violent. Even a simple handshake that is too firm can be uncomfortable instead of being reassuring.

The psychological dimension of touch tells you that though all forms of contact stem from the same physiological process, you perceive them differently on the basis of your own emotions for the person who reaches out for you; the feelings of the person who offers the touch; or a combination of both these situations. In other words, the healing caress of a mother (vis-à-vis her child) is not the same as a friendly pat from a colleague, and neither of these can be compared to the way in which an individual touches her/his lover.

With partner yoga, touch is the most important 'ingredient' for communication; indeed, it is the very language. Even without words, your body will reveal your intent, and a touch can highlight your feelings, make evident to your companion what it is that makes you happy or anxious or calm. As you advance in the practice of partner yoga, your companion and you will be able to understand each other through touch, and the need to exchange verbal commands will progressively diminish. The same asana will take a different meaning once you establish this form of connection with your collaborator.

Do You Know These Curious Facts about Touch?

› Touch stimulates the brain to release endorphins (the body's natural painkillers).
› Blood pressure and the heart rate can be reduced even by a simple touch.
› There are approximately five million touch receptors in the skin—3,000 of which are on one fingertip.
› Among the body's most sensitive areas are the lips, the back of the neck, the fingertips and the soles of the feet. The least sensitive area is the middle of your back.
› Being touched can reduce stress, by lowering levels of hormones like cortisol.
› Pain is the body's warning system and it's thorough. People have more receptors for pain than for any other sensation.
› Whiskers, which have tactile sense, are used by animals for a number of purposes, including navigation, detecting water currents and texture discrimination.
› Grasshoppers have hair all over the outside of their bodies to detect air movement.

TRUST ME:
THE VALUE OF PARTNER YOGA

In everyday life, there are several situations when we seek the support of others—be it when we desperately need advice, or simply want someone to laugh with over a joke. We all have felt the power of a connected relationship, and indeed, yearn for it. Yoga operates within this principle, and to enhance yogic practice, one of the best things we can do is involve another individual. Suddenly, the experience and the perception of the asana changes, and we see and feel things that we had never sensed before. We get to stretch the limits of postures in ways we never thought was possible.

Getting into an asana with a partner challenges us both physically and emotionally. We are coerced to exit our comfort zone, as we have to get accustomed to placing our bodies in another's hands, quite literally. One could say that partner yoga is an accelerated means of experiencing the key principle of yoga—union.

While partner yoga is not a substitute for individual practice, it does build on it, while also incorporating the element of touch and the presence of another person to deepen the impact of a posture. Such poses are not merely variations of existing individual asanas, but are entirely new, so to speak. While practising them, we have to make the mental shift from rigidly expecting postures to mirror solo asanas, to enthusiastically exploring new possibilities, new challenges, new and entertaining ways of approaching a yoga mat.

AWARENESS

Partner yoga allows you to deepen your self-awareness. In your partner, you have a mirror, a physical presence who sheds light on your disposition. By collaborating and performing asanas as one, your behaviour patterns, thoughts and feelings come to the fore and you get to explore your inner life in ways that you would find difficult on a busy working day.

Equally, since partners reflect the attitudes you project on them, partner yoga helps you enhance your alertness to the 'other'. Moreover, the way you interact during a partner yoga session can provide insights into the way you relate to one another under normal circumstances. As the two of you support each other, while focusing on movement, play, breath and intimacy, a context is created for examining the larger principles that steer the association.

Practising together obliges you to be involved with one another, and *listen* to gain useful insights into communicating without words. You get to observe who takes control and how, who gives in and why, who trusts and who doesn't.

In a wider context, you get to see where you belong on the social spectrum—whether you put others' well-being before your own and deprive yourself; or maintain a strict distance to avoid disillusionment. Between these two extreme personality types, partner yoga helps you understand where you can place yourself as a social being.

INTERDEPENDENCE, VULNERABILITY AND TRUST-BUILDING

Many of us believe that our goals (including our yogic practice) can be best pursued when we operate alone; dealing with the needs and feelings of someone else is an additional burden and complication that can be avoided. Partner yoga upends this notion, by revealing that we can accomplish much more when we (willingly) support one another.

Consequently, this form of yoga highlights our interdependence. While we may think of ourselves as self-sufficient creatures, practising yoga with another person can remind us of the vital need to reach out, and also the beauty and freedom intrinsic to any healthy association.

Moreover, partner yoga reinforces the fact that cooperation and interdependence are linked. Postures in partner yoga hinge on two people showing up, exerting the same kind of effort, and working, not as individuals, but as a team, keeping their differences at bay and aiming for a common goal.

Partner yoga makes us accept our vulnerabilities in the presence of another person. Equally, the support we require from a partner to enter an asana and maintain it will inevitably shatter our views regarding a separate self/ego (which, ironically, is that part of us that suffers the pain of loneliness while we cling to the illusion of independence).

Even though your companion and you cannot see each other while bending or twisting in an asana, you know that you are connected with one another and can feel each other's strength. When you attempt a partner yoga pose, you need to trust in your collaborator's capacity and readiness to help, protect and respect your body, and s/he has to believe in you. Trust is the core of any relationship—if there is no trust, there is no meaning to an association—and partner yoga strengthens your capacity to offer and receive this gift.

Finally, once you achieve the desired pose, you not only feel confident about yourself, but also about your relationship with your partner—which has got you to this point of accomplishment.

INTIMACY

While not specifically designed for lovers, partner yoga can be a tool to build intimacy and deepen a bond, even while working out, stretching, balancing and meditating.

If you are practising with a friend, you will have the opportunity to make your association deeper and richer, marked by openness and honesty. The connection you establish will be non-verbal, and therefore, more authentic, suffused with compassion for each other's mistakes. Beyond the yoga mat, in the real world, you'll find your friendship only strengthening after partner yoga.

In the specific case of lovers, partner yoga can help the couple bridge any divide in their relationship, be it physical, emotional or psychological. Practising with your lover will inevitably bring you closer to her/him. After all, maintaining the right balance and alignment, remaining focused on posture while the eyes are closed and listening to each other's breath for cues, requires an emotional and mental cooperation; after a session, you'll inevitably discover that your empathy for your partner has increased.

Partner yoga can be particularly beneficial for those battling sexual issues. This is especially true for those with lifestyles that grant little time for intimacy; partner yoga—gentle and slow—helps lovers depart from their usual workaday roles, rely on each other, embrace their sensuality and build a subtle erotic connectedness. They also become aware of a lover's reactions, which can offer signposts beyond the yoga mat.

HAPPINESS

Your body and mind are connected and work together. With regular yoga practice, your body gains in strength and flexibility, and develops greater control, which grants you a sense of well-being. Partner yoga enhances this feeling, not just at the physical, but at the psychological level, too.

The happiness within relationships is linked to the degree to which partners pay attention to and enjoy one another's presence. This can't happen through force or manipulation; it has to happen naturally, with ease and delight. Partner yoga facilitates the process.

THE PARTNERS IN
PARTNER YOGA

TEAM MOMMY:
YOGA FOR MOTHER AND CHILD

Partner yoga, as we've established, is not just for lovers. Nor is it inextricably linked to sensuality or sexuality. Rather, it works within the framework of all associations, intimate or platonic, formal or informal. Since there is probably no relationship more profound and enigmatic than that between a mother and her offspring, it's not surprising that partner yoga finds relevance in this context, too.

■

A pregnant woman is likely to go through a rollercoaster of emotions—from excitement and anxiety in the first trimester, to joyous anticipation in the third trimester when she begins to understand her baby a lot better.

Physically, throughout pregnancy, a mother's body goes through a whole lot of stress due to hormonal changes. There's a sudden and dramatic increase in oestrogen—more than will ever be experienced at any other point in a lifetime—which allows the placenta to transfer nutrients, and the uterus to support the developing baby. There's also a massive rise in progesterone, which leads to a loosening of ligaments, tendons and joints across the body, and makes the uterus transform from a small pear-sized organ to one that can accommodate a full-term baby.

During pregnancy, a woman's posture changes, with the abdomen becoming convex, and the curve of the back growing more intense, all of which leads to a shift in the centre of gravity. Equally, while expecting, a woman can gain considerable weight; among other things, this slows the circulation of blood, particularly to the lower limbs, and leads to a retention of fluids and the swelling of the feet, legs and hands.

Given the spate and the intensity of physical changes, it takes time for a mother's body to return to its pre-pregnancy state post-delivery. When a new mother leaves the hospital, she may still 'look' as though she's expecting; her abdominal muscles may be stretched and untoned, and her skin may sag. This could be trying for her.

In addition, the dramatic lifestyle changes that come with early parenthood—sleepless nights, breastfeeding and care of the baby— and the specific challenges that confront new mothers—the baby may not attach herself to the breast or may keep odd hours—can make this special phase in a woman's life somewhat nerve-wracking.

In these times of anxiety, one is reminded of a Persian saying: 'Children are the bridge to heaven'. Yet how is a new mother to experience the joys of maternity, the fulfilment that comes with child-rearing, when she is tense?

■

One of the most effective tools for de-stressing can be yoga. For a mother—who would like to practise yoga but cannot spend a long time away from her baby—there are variations that involve her child.

The structure and length of yoga poses for a mother and child are unlike those of regular 'partner yoga'. After all, if mothers are practising yoga with babies or toddlers, they have to deal with breastfeeding breaks, diaper-changing sessions and the little one's unpredictable mood-swings.

Consequently, while practising yoga with a child, it's important for moms to remember that the asanas may not be as beautiful or graceful as pictures make them out to be. But that hardly matters! The emphasis is tapping into the essence of yogic practice—which is bonding—rather than achieving choreographed performances.

Practising with children can be fun—for, kids are more flexible than adults, come without preconceived notions and are generally adventurous. Being good mimics, they can mirror the mother's asanas quite easily and learn quickly. Moreover, since children tend to focus on any activity that they find interesting and enjoyable, mothers find that with a little creativity—by associating asanas, for instance, with animals or playful shapes and objects— their offspring need little encouragement to practise yoga!

At times, it is also important for a mom to allow her little girl (or boy) to lead the class. All she needs to do is put her on the mat, sit in front of her, and mirror what she is doing—rolling on the floor, crawling to the other end of the room, or kicking the legs in the air. It may sound bizarre at first, but soon the new mom will lose her inhibitions and feel as though she is becoming a child; this will help her reach a place of mutual understanding with her offspring, while also allowing her child to see her—the authoritative parent—from a wholly different perspective!

It goes without saying that mother and child partner yoga can also be practised by father and child. Indeed, kids, with their infectious energy, make reluctant fathers feel so comfortable that they ungrudgingly attempt partner yoga!

Partner yoga with one's offspring can be a very rewarding way of spending time as a family—especially today, when parents are often obliged to resume their professional careers soon after a child's birth, and find 'quality time' a scarce commodity.

■

If partner yoga for mother and child is special, it's because it lets Mom gift her baby her 'healing touch'. Dr Marshal Klaus, a neonatologist, and Dr John Kennell, a paediatrician, coined the term 'bonding' in the 1970s to describe the marvel of a mother falling in love with her baby if both had skin contact for thirty to sixty minutes after the child's birth. Indeed, this is the beginning of motherly love.

A mother's touch stimulates breathing in the new-born, and her heartbeat can quieten the baby who is used to the uterine environment. At the same time, the mother stands to benefit from such interaction. Nipple contact encourages the release of oxytocin, the so-called 'cuddle hormone', which not only heightens maternal feelings but also helps the uterus contract.

Studies show that a baby's heart beats just a little faster at the sound of the mother's voice. What else is this but a synchronized dance of physiologies? Mother–child partner yoga only makes such miracles more commonplace!

THE BENEFITS OF MOTHER–CHILD PARTNER YOGA FOR THE YOUNG 'UN

Mother–child partner yoga is a shared experience that encourages early bonding patterns in children. Besides creating conditions that foster an overall sense of well-being, it also promotes normal, healthy growth in kids and prevents later developmental problems.

Indeed, each movement that constitutes mother–child partner yoga supports the offspring's growth—strengthening the physical body, maintaining flexibility, developing a healthy posture, improving coordination and alleviating early health issues. The massage provided by the mother to her offspring during practice sessions aids digestion, thereby giving relief to a child who is colicky. Equally, tactile stimulation, which is part and parcel of such yoga, not only contributes to the development of a child's brain and nervous system, but also makes her relax; baby yoga, with movements that mimic the soothing rocking that a foetus experiences in the womb, has long been known to calm energetic children and improve sleep patterns.

Most significantly, this form of partner yoga is educational and plants the seeds of a future of yogic practice and meditation

What is Kangaroo Care?

Kangaroo care is a method of holding a baby that involves skin-to-skin contact. The baby, who is naked (except for a diaper and a piece of cloth covering the back), is placed in an upright position against a parent's bare chest. This snuggling of the infant inside the piece of cloth in proximity to the parent's body—much like a joey in a kangaroo's pouch—has led to the term 'kangaroo care'.

Kangaroo care emerged in response to the mind-bogglingly high death rate of 70 per cent among pre-term babies, due to infections, respiratory problems and so on, in Bogota, Columbia in the late 1970s. Researchers found that babies held close to their mothers' bodies for large portions of the day, not only survived, but also thrived. In the United States, hospitals that encourage kangaroo care typically have mothers or fathers providing skin-to-skin contact to their pre-term babies for several hours each day.

Kangaroo care benefits the baby in the following ways. It ensures:

- › The stabilization of the baby's heart rate
- › Improved (more regular) breathing patterns
- › Improved oxygen saturation levels (an indicator of how well oxygen is being delivered to all the infant's organs and tissues)
- › An increase in sleep time
- › More rapid weight gain
- › Contentment, with fewer instances of crying
- › More successful breastfeeding episodes
- › Earlier hospital discharge

Kangaroo care benefits parents in the following ways. It leads to:

- › Improved bonding and feelings of tenderness towards the baby
- › A greater supply of breast milk
- › More confidence about the ability to tend to the baby
- › Greater conviction that the baby is well-cared for
- › An enhanced sense of control

in children. Watching Mom or Dad practise yoga with them has a positive impact on the choices kids make and ensures that they take care of themselves when they grow older. They also learn an important value early on: humility. As mother–child partner yoga makes children aware of their bodies—its wonderful strengths and its limitations—they learn to accept themselves as they are, and forgive not only their own 'failings', but also the physical limitations of the partner (in this case, the parent).

THE BENEFITS OF MOTHER–CHILD PARTNER YOGA FOR THE NEW MOM

Partner yoga helps the mother—who begins developing a strong maternal bond when her baby is in the womb—strengthen her relationship with her offspring, cement it with compassion and empathy, while also bringing the family close. Besides, it takes the association to a territory where there are no contradictory pulls as both enter each other's mental and physical spaces.

Practising this form of yoga is fun—it makes Mom and baby happy; it makes them giggle. It relaxes an overwrought mother, and fosters self-awareness and self-confidence in someone who is edgy and unsure. Additionally, mother–child partner yoga improves a mom's imagination, as she has to improvise with asanas, and find ways of practising them while keeping the weight, height and strength of her child in mind.

Then, there are huge physical benefits. Through regular practice, a mother is able to recover from the rigours of pregnancy by reclaiming her body, flexing her muscles and gently stretching her joints. She begins regaining her strength, shedding those extra pounds and attaining a toned body after delivery. In particular, the asana sequences performed with her child help her build and tone her abdominal and pelvic floor muscles.

ASANAS FOR MOTHER AND CHILD

In this book, you will find an asana-bank, with detailed instructions and tips for the execution of a series of postures that can be practised by partners. While these may work within the context of most associations—friends or colleagues or lovers—they have to be adapted to fit the needs of a mother and child.

As an early compass, a few variations of standard asanas have been listed below, so Mom and baby can practise together.

Asana 1: Touch, Breathe and Connect

This is a simple exercise that will help you (the mother) establish a connection with your baby. The touch of your hand on the baby's belly and the synchronization of your breaths can be soothing and comforting for both of you.

Method

1. Sit in a comfortable position, with your baby lying on her back in front of you.
2. Place one hand on your own tummy and one hand on your baby's tummy. As you look into your baby's eyes, notice how she breathes, and observe the movement of her belly.
3. Mimic your baby's belly breathing. As you inhale, breathe into your hand. As you exhale, draw your navel towards your spine and lift your pelvic floor muscles.
4. Repeat this multiple times.

Asana 2: The Flying Little Yogi

Your baby will enjoy this asana as much as she likes levitating (and which baby doesn't?). For you, this asana is a means of relaxing, as also toning your body.

Method

1. Lie down on your back with your baby on your chest.
2. Slowly bend your knees and bring them close to your chest. Gently place your baby securely on your shins, with the baby's tummy down.
3. Look into your baby's eyes while you keep your hands wrapped around her back to keep her secure.
4. Bring your head and shoulders towards your baby, activating your abdominal muscles as you release your breath; lift your head high enough to touch your nose to the tip of the baby's.
5. Gently lower your head and place it back on the mat. Draw your knees in, bringing them close to your chest, to curl your lower back.
6. Hold on for four long and deep breaths, then four slow breaths. Gently move your feet up and down to watch your baby giggle. Maintain eye contact with the baby. Repeat as often as you like.

Asana 3: The Downward-facing Dog and the Baby

This asana is a lot of fun for your baby, as she will love the element of surprise it comes with! You can even play peek-a-boo. For you, this asana is hugely beneficial since it eases the tightness in your back and neck, and provides a gentle massage to the shoulders and the tummy.

Method

1. Start by standing on your knees. The baby lies in front of you with her belly facing up.
2. Bend towards your baby. Align your palms directly under your shoulders and your knees beneath your hips. Your baby is now underneath you with her head below your face.
3. Spread your fingers wide on the mat to have a firm grip.

Point your toes inward and gently lift your knees off the mat. This brings you into the downward-facing dog pose, or adho mukha svanasana/parvatasana (asana 12 under 'the preparatory series'). In other words, you now hold 'an upside-down V' posture.

4. Keep your eyes open and look into your baby's eyes as you hold this asana. Breathe in and out, with slow and comfortable breaths.

5. Breathe in and push your body forward, assuming the plank pose (in other words, your body is in one line from the top of your head to your heels; your head is a natural extension of your spine; your heels point towards the ceiling and your palms are flat). Do not dip or raise your hips. Repeat this a couple of times. Your baby will love it as you come up close from a distance.

Asana 4: The Shadow

This asana is a lot of fun. But it's also very challenging, since babies are known to be flexible. Are you nimble enough to nibble your own big toe?

Method

1. Simply seat your baby right in front of you.
2. Watch your baby move and mirror these actions.
3. Do this as long as you can.

If your child has a lot of energy and refuses to sit or lie down in any position for more than a few seconds, do not worry or get exasperated. Forget conventional asana wisdom and accept the baby's moves as your personal yogic posture flow.

WORKDAY WORKOUT:
YOGA AMONG COLLEAGUES

O f all the forms of exercise, yoga at the workplace is the most convenient. It can be practised within a fairly small office, with minimal equipment, and each individual, no matter her/his body type, can participate.

When corporate yoga assumes the form of partner yoga, the results can be stunning. Not only do employees experience health benefits but they also build solid bonds with one another—work-mates now become yoga buddies! At any point of the working day, a yoga break can be arranged; employees, thus, get involved with a relaxing, nourishing and challenging session that also gets the adrenaline pumping.

THE BENEFITS OF PARTNER YOGA WITH COLLEAGUES

To begin with, partner yoga in the office gifts you the break you so badly need from your desk and your work! You get to ditch your sedentary position and move your body. You also get to focus your thoughts on something other than schedules, appointments and sales figures! The mind gets some much-needed rest, your soul is recharged and your limbs get the workout they have been craving—this might, in fact, be the only opportunity for exercise they have been afforded in weeks! Suddenly, you have a spring in your step!

Partner yoga at the workplace helps you establish a connection or 'break the ice' with people you would otherwise share most of your workday with, without moving beyond regular 'office chit-chat'. It may also be the only time you liaise with colleagues across different departments.

Through this form of partner yoga—which brings colleagues together under circumstances where they need to rely on one another for support—office hierarchies are erased and participants are freed from restrictive roles and positions. In the case of those who are senior, it helps them transcend their egos, if any. In the case of junior employees, it helps them discover the true personalities of their team leaders, which makes working with them easier and much more fun; they get to move past preconceived notions, many of which emerge during staff meetings or formal interactions. In fact, since several asanas come with unusual positions, one partner inevitably breaks out laughing. This instantly creates a relaxed environment, and encourages casual conversation.

As with any form of yoga, partner yoga among colleagues helps you discover your own physical limits, mental stamina and endurance levels. But in addition, this form of practice makes you understand a co-worker's strengths and weaknesses, and surmount all blind spots in the spirit of cooperation.

Equally, partner yoga among colleagues—which compels you to explore ways of interaction that go beyond verbal communication—helps you fine-tune your sensitivity to a co-worker. Slowly, as you make the adjustments required to maintain your own balance, yet support your workfellow, relying on nothing more than a smile or the push-and-pull of your body, you begin liaising in a positive, rather than in a highly competitive space.

Yoga, in general, is calming and eases stress. In the context of partner yoga, the moment you let go and allow a colleague to share the responsibility of completing an asana and making it stable, you not only learn a vital life-lesson—not everything depends on you!—but you can also sense your anxieties wash away. As you shift your awareness to the flow of breath, the mind calms.

This form of partner yoga (like others) builds trust. Some asanas, which are fairly advanced, may require one co-worker to hang from the body of the other in an inverted position, or might make a colleague bear the weight of another. None of this will be possible without faith in the capacity of one's 'yoga buddy' to keep one safe and secure.

Now, why should any of this matter within an organization? Well, because what happens on the yoga mat influences every interaction outside. The cooperation, trust and camaraderie that is developed during practice sessions, immediately translates into better workplace dynamics. As you get to know your colleagues, share laughs and surmount challenges on the yoga mat, you find yourself, as an employee, transforming! You get to be yourself without crippling inhibitions, flaunt your creativity without fearing ridicule, communicate openly without being encumbered by 'protocol', cooperate without feeling threatened, and lend a hand without passing judgement. What this means is that within an organization, information flows freely, projects get completed beautifully, productivity improves (as things get done with lightning speed!), and the company, as a whole, becomes balanced, functional and successful.

Some asanas that work wonderfully in an office environment include the 'blooming pose' (asana 14 under 'partner yoga') and 'sit together pose' (asana 15 under 'partner yoga'). Completing (or even attempting) these postures equip you with skills that are very relevant to office management. You learn to go the extra mile, take ownership of tasks and work through problems.

LOVE ALL:
YOGA FOR COUPLES

Couple's yoga builds the most holistic bond conceivable between two people since it encompasses the physical (touch), the emotional (understanding and trust) and the spiritual (intimacy). It blends all the elements of mother–child and colleagues' yoga, and then adds a little extra magic!

To understand how partner yoga benefits a couple, we can draw a parallel with 'koshas'—the layer of existence described in Vedantic philosophy (more about this soon)—and the principle that 'three bodies' define every human being.

You read that right. According to Vedantic and yogic philosophy, you have more than just one body. The first, which is the most familiar to you, is the 'physical body'—made of flesh and bones—which takes birth, grows, decays and finally, dies. The second is the 'astral or subtle body', which includes the five organs of action/movement (the mouth, hands, feet, anus and genitals); prana (breath); the mind (that feels and doubts); the intellect (that analyses and discerns); the subconscious (that stores memories) and the ego (the self-assertive principle). The third body—the so-called 'causal body'—contains the impressions left by all the experiences of this life and beyond. It is where the soul rests in a deep state of sleep while still ignorant about being part of the divine.

KOSHAS

Emerging from the Sanskrit word for 'sheath', koshas are described in Vedantic philosophy as the layers that make human existence—

often compared to the whorls of an onion. These layers move from the outermost realm of the physical to the deep spiritual core of the individual soul.

Kosha layers do not exist purely in the spiritual dimension— they come with their own specific physiological functions and psychological underpinnings. In fact, one is constantly interacting with koshas without even being fully aware of this!

Let's take a brief journey through koshas to understand them better.

What is Vedanta?

Vedanta is one of the six orthodox schools of Hindu philosophy. The term 'Veda' means 'knowledge' and 'anta' means 'end'; it is, therefore, considered the last of the Vedic revelations. The three main texts around which Vedanta revolves are the Upanishads, the Brahma Sutras and the Bhagavad Gita.

Vedanta explores the relation between the individual soul (jiva-atman) and the Supreme Being or Universal Soul (Brahman). In fact, by its yardstick, Brahman is the only reality; the world is an illusion. And we are beings who end up believing in the existence of the world thanks to the illusory powers of Brahman, called Maya.

Our ignorance of this chimerical world is what causes all suffering. Only when we realize a true understanding of Brahman can we attain liberation from pain. Liberation, in other words, lies in knowing the reality of the non-difference (advaita or 'non-duality') between one's soul and God.

Annamaya Kosha

The first of all koshas and the outermost layer is described as the 'food sheath'. It acknowledges the physical needs of the body (such as a good meal), and represents the body (including the skin, muscles, connective tissue, fat and bones). Place your hand on your knees and feel the skin and bones—you are now engaging with the annamaya kosha. In fact, a lot of people are *entirely* absorbed by this 'layer of being'—for, they spend most of their time indulging the physical senses. This is observed when two lovers become slaves of gastronomical pleasures or are held in thrall of sensual delights.

On another note: Why is the first layer—that revolves around the physical body—referred to as the food sheath? It's because, according to yogic philosophy, a newborn's body is nurtured by mother's milk; the adult body grows with the intake of food; and at the end, the aged body, once dead, becomes nourishment for other creatures. Hence, the physical being is no more than a minuscule part of a food chain. It is also non-eternal, subject to disease and decay (unlike the soul that it cages within).

Pranamaya Kosha

The second layer is the one that keeps you alive—for, it's linked to 'prana', or vital energy. The Sanskrit word 'prana' is a compound of 'pra', which means 'prior' or 'to have a previous existence', and 'ana', which refers to a basic element that lies at the very foundation of everything. So the word 'prana' literally implies 'that which is a prerequisite to life'. It is precisely this 'life-giving force' which shapes the world; prana is energy.

Besides being concerned with breath and the flow of such vital energy through the physical being, this kosha also includes the fluid, physical aspects of the anatomical body—the circulation of blood and the movement of lymph and cerebrospinal fluids. In psychological terms, the pranamaya kosha controls the rhythm of the body and the spirit.

Manomaya Kosha

While modern science has developed an acute understanding of the inner workings of the brain, motivations and emotions still retain a mysterious quality. The third layer, then, takes you into the deep recesses of the mind and the nervous system; it acts as the control panel that links the emotional core and the physical body, sending messages back and forth. Manomaya kosha is the layer where human instincts reside (for instance, reactions to potential danger, survival skills, sexual desire and so on). At this layer, every human being is alike.

Vijanamaya Kosha

On diving beneath the sea of emotions, you chance upon the fourth kosha—vijanamaya—the knowledge sheath or the layer of the intellect. Composed of all the wisdom and awareness you have gained over time, it is this layer that helps you further develop your sagacity and astuteness. Unlike the previous koshas, at this layer every human being is unique, as everyone's path to knowledge is marked by specific individual experiences. Moreover, it is when this kosha operates that a couple (or any two individuals) can enjoy a conversation with each other in a spirit of openness.

Anandamaya Kosha

The fifth and last kosha drops from conscious awareness to the pure and radiant 'bliss body'. When you sink into the anandamaya kosha, you could well experience a connection with all things, a sense of liberation from suffering and a state of just *being*—often described as 'in the flow'. You are in harmony with yourself and the environment you are in. This translates into a new level of joy and love in your relationships.

∎

If partner yoga is done with the right intention—with a mindset of openness; with an attitude of forgiveness and acceptance of one's own and one's partner's limitations and imperfections; with the willingness to experiment with dynamics and roles—it can be extremely beneficial to couples. With partner yoga, lovers can bridge any disconnect and build a perfect, problem-free connection. This can be understood even better by considering koshas intimately.

ANNAMAYA KOSHA AND COUPLE'S YOGA

Imagine that each partner is like a building with five storeys. At every floor, a bridge is erected to connect the two structures. Now, let's call the ground floor 'annamaya kosha', and the bridge connecting the two buildings (that is, partners) here is composed of asanas. Couples work at the level of the annamaya kosha when they perform asanas individually, as well as together (in partner yoga).

There's no escaping the first of all koshas. If the primary aim of yoga (as mentioned in the introductory chapter) is to establish a union between the individual soul (jiva-atma) and the universal (param-atma) through a state of deep meditation, one has to *first* develop physical and mental strength and focus—so as to hold a stable and comfortable meditative position without being plagued by an aching body or a wandering mind. Indeed, in his classical text, Yoga Sutra, Patanjali himself said that an asana must be 'sukham' (comfortable), 'sthiram' (steady), 'asanam' (meditative).

In other words, before entering the spiritual dimension, a steady and comfortable position is key to experiencing the many benefits of yoga. When your breath flows calmly and deeply through your twisted, bent or stretched body; when your senses remain sharp and your awareness is rooted in the present moment; when your body and your mind are quiet—only then can you become aware of koshas.

In fact, you see a beautiful circle emerging, while you are holding an asana. When you focus on your breath, you essentially concentrate on inhaling, exhaling and calming your mind, while cultivating awareness. Once you're aware, you understand your body better; instead of pushing your body into an asana, you work towards letting the asana become one with your body, respecting your flexibility, strength and stability. As a result, you will no longer struggle in a posture, but will hold it with greater ease and comfort. Your mind, therefore, becomes as clear as water, as calm as a pool.

While practising couple's yoga, when trying to reach a level of comfort, the two practitioners need to balance their weight, remain sensitive to the push-and-pull of two bodies, and distribute their combined strength, while acknowledging any kind of resistance. This joint physical effort sees the couple interacting and communicating at the level of the annamaya kosha.

PRANAMAYA KOSHA AND COUPLE'S YOGA

As human beings, we receive 'life-giving' prana most abundantly through the air we breathe. But prana is also in the food we eat and the water we drink. Believe it or not, touch, too, can be charged with prana and transferred to another person through a warm hug or a firm handshake.

The last point becomes especially relevant in the context of couple's yoga. While practising this form of yoga, the regulation of prana within the individual body transforms into the regulation of prana between two bodies, as energy flows from one to the next— establishing an energy-rich form of communication that unites a couple into one pranic entity. To nudge the metaphor used earlier, you are now in the second floor of your individual buildings—the bridge that unites the two structures is composed of prana.

But how is prana to be regulated? Quite simply, through pranayama—the yogic technique of controlling breath, and fine-tuning inhalation and exhalation (imperative, as most of us breathe poorly and extract insufficient prana). In truth, pranayama translates into more than just breathing exercises. Through pranayama, a practitioner, after mastering breath control, progressively manages to control the flow of thoughts on the mat, and ultimately takes charge of the mind.

Pranayama

Pranayama is a very complex discipline that requires constant and consistent practice to be mastered. Given how potent it is, ensure that you practise it only under the supervision of a trained teacher, to avoid any kind of health risk.

All pranayama exercises, performed individually or as part of a couple, are to be performed in a comfortable cross-legged, seated position, with the spine straight, shoulders relaxed and eyes gently closed, so as to focus all attention inwards. In this context, two key exercises are listed below.

Anuloma Viloma

1. Place your right hand in the Vishnu mudra—with the index and middle fingers bent towards the palm of the hand and the other fingers straight.
2. Exhale completely and, keeping the right hand in the Vishnu mudra, close your right nostril with your right thumb. Inhale from the left nostril at the count of four. Close your left nostril with the two end fingers of your right hand in the Vishnu mudra and retain your breath to the count of sixteen.
3. Release the right thumb from your right nostril and exhale through it at the count of eight.
4. Inhale from the right nostril, retain your breath and exhale from the left nostril, retaining the count of four-sixteen-eight. This completes one round.
5. Repeat this for ten rounds.

If your nasal passages are clear, the breath naturally alternates between the two nostrils. This alternate breathing exercise lends balance to your breathing and nostril dominance patterns. It also balances both the hemispheres of the brain by stimulating them equally.

Bhastrika

To perform this exercise, you have to inhale and exhale rapidly, activating the diaphragm and the intercostal muscles. Bhastrika is said to have a powerful cleansing effect. It is, therefore, a good preparatory exercise for chakra meditation (more about this later).

Nadis

Now, let's delve deeper into the term, 'prana'. Prana is akin to an electrical charge that runs within the body through 'nadis'. In yogic tradition, a nadi is like a channel that transports prana all over the body, in the same way that the veins transport blood.

According to tantric philosophy (more about this soon), there are 72,000 or more 'nadis' or 'channels' within the human body through which the electric current that is prana flows from one point to the next. For prana to flow smoothly, it is important for nadis to function well, and to remain clear of obstructions that can block energy.

Among these 72,000 nadis, three are particularly important. Let's begin with sushumna—the central nadi that corresponds to the spinal column. The two nadis on either side of sushumna are known as ida and pingala. The ida and pingala nadis are often viewed as reflections of the two hemispheres of the brain, and are respectively, said to correspond to the left and right sympathetic nervous cords in the physical body.

Pingala—which means 'tawny' in Sanskrit—is associated with the sun. It's male energy and in terms of temperature is (expectedly) hot. Ida, on the other hand—which means 'comfort' in Sanskrit—is associated with the moon. It is female energy and has a cooling effect.

Ida and pingala are believed to be stimulated through different pranayama practices, including alternate breathing through the left and right nostrils (to stimulate the left and right sides of the brain by turns). Sushumna, on its part, helps both nostrils remain open and free for the passage of air.

What is Tantra?

The term 'tantra' (or 'tantrism') is linked to a large number of texts and rituals practised by Hindu, Buddhist and Jain communities in South and East Asia from the fifth century.

According to tantric philosophy, the world we see and experience is a concrete manifestation of divine energy. In order to liberate oneself spiritually and unite with the divine, one needs to ritually master and channel energy. By doing this, besides attaining spiritual insight, an individual will be able to attain 'worldly' benefits, such as wealth, fame and even supernatural skills.

According to Hindu tantric tradition, the energy that creates, sustains and destroys the universe is known as Shakti. Goddess Shakti is represented in an ecstatic union with her consort: the Hindu god, Shiva, who represents consciousness. Shiva and Shakti, consciousness and energy, are two sides of the same coin. Energy without consciousness is aimless and lacks direction. On the other hand, consciousness without energy is inactive and cannot make anything happen.

Tantra has influenced many non-tantric traditions in Hindu philosophy, including hatha yoga. However, the tantric approach remains profoundly different from the other schools of thought. For instance, while Patanjali viewed spirituality as distinct from the everyday world (suggesting that one should withdraw from sensual pleasure to quieten the mind and access the divine), tantrism sees the body and the material aspects of life as manifestations of the divine. It sees the body as a vehicle that, through worldly experiences, attains liberation.

∎

Tantra, as synonymous with esoteric sexual practices, is a modern-day misconception. In its purest form, tantric philosophy is far removed from free love! In some tantric traditions, sexual union (maithuna) was viewed as one of the possible means of awakening and mastering Shakti. But this practice was rarely followed and was restricted to highly controlled esoteric rituals. Moreover, it was never employed without warning, to prevent any possibility of its abuse.

Tantrism's identification with sex is linked to the misunderstanding that the Kamasutra is a tantric text. However, this is an entirely false assumption: while tantra (as we now know) is a philosophical tenet that proposes a path towards the divine, the Kamasutra is a 'manual' of ancient times to help people perform their duties while also enjoying the good things of the world. In fact, the Kamasutra is based on an even older text titled Kama Shastra, which along with the Artha Shastra and the Dharma Shastra, sheds light on the aims of life.

Chakras

The key points of intersection of the nadis are known as 'chakras'. 'Chakra' is derived from the Sanskrit word 'wheel'; if translated literally it means 'wheel of spinning energy'. This isn't a poor word-picture, for a chakra is actually a whirling, vortex-like powerhouse!

We have seven main chakras (and many more minor ones) in the body. To visualize them, imagine a vertical power current that runs up and down the spine (or sushumna, the central nadi in the astral body), from the top of the head to the base of the cord. The seven major chakras are aligned with this vertical 'power line'.

Chakras connect your astral body to your physical one. Sometimes they can even get blocked because of stress, emotional upheaval or physical problems. If the body's energy system cannot flow freely, you find yourself remaining physically frail or feeling mentally and emotionally out of sync.

So what are the seven power centres that can positively affect our sense of well-being? Let's consider them in reverse order.

Chakra 7: Sahasrara

Also known as the crown chakra, sahasrara is linked to a state of pure consciousness—so there is neither object nor subject. When kundalini energy (Shakti) rises to this point, it unites with male Shiva energy, and a state of intense concentration is attained.

In other words, sahasrara is associated with divine purpose and personal destiny, and hones understanding, acceptance and bliss.

This chakra is represented by the colour violet, and is located at the top of the head. It is associated with the cerebral cortex, central nervous system and the pituitary gland.

Chakra 6: Ajna

Also known as the third eye, ajna balances the higher and lower selves, provides inner guidance and offers pure clarity at an intuitive level.

This chakra hones perception, intuition and wisdom; dreams, intuitions, wishes and recollections are held within ajna.

This chakra is represented by the colour indigo (a combination of red and blue), and is located in the centre of the forehead, slightly above eye level. It is associated with the sensitive pineal gland, which produces the hormone melatonin that regulates sleep, as also (according to Dr Rick Strassman) the psychedelic chemical dimethyltryptamine—the only known hallucinogen endogenous to the human body.

Chakra 5: Vishuddha

Also known as the throat chakra, vishuddha is associated with the element of ether, and is linked to communication and growth through expression.

Vishuddha hones self-expression, creativity and judgement.

This chakra is represented through the colour blue or turquoise, and is located parallel to the thyroid gland—which produces a hormone responsible for growth and maturation—as also, at a more general level, the neck, shoulders, arms, hands and parathyroid glands.

Chakra 4: Anahata

Also known as the heart chakra, anahata is associated with the element of air and covers the gamut of fairly complex emotions—compassion, unconditional love, a sense of rejection or well-being.

Anahata hones love for the self and for others, harmony and peace.

This chakra is represented through the colours green or pink, and corresponds with the thymus in the chest—the site of the maturation of T-cells, responsible for fending off diseases—as also, at a more general level, the lungs and heart.

Chakra 3: Manipura

Also known as the navel chakra, manipura is associated with the element of fire. It is the seat of one's emotional life—governing feelings of personal power, joy and anger. Besides, sensitivity, ambition and the ability to achieve are also stored here.

Manipura hones vital life-skills like opinion-formation; helps manage fear and anxiety; and makes one advance from base emotions to more holistic ones.

This chakra is represented through the colour yellow, and is believed to correspond to the pancreas, as well as the outer adrenal glands and the adrenal cortex (that play a valuable role in digestion and converting food into energy).

Chakra 2: Svadhishthana

Also known as the sacral chakra, svadhishthana is associated with the element of water. It governs not only reproduction, but also creativity and enthusiasm. This chakra steers the two big Ps: pleasure and procreation.

You now see the mighty pieces of this puzzle fall into place: you fall in love through the anahata/heart chakra; this feeling of unconditional love moves to the manipura chakra/ the emotional centre; when these energies transition to svadhishthana, you experience the urge to marry, settle down or build a more permanent association.

The svadhishthana chakra is represented through the colour orange. Located in the sacrum, it is said to correspond to the testes or the ovaries (that produce sex hormones), as well as, at a more general level, to the genito-urinary system, including the kidneys and bladder.

Chakra 1: Muladhara

Also known as the root chakra, muladhara is associated with the element of earth, since it is closest to terra firma. It is also for this reason that it is linked to the 'grounding' principles of physical survival, such as the fight-or-flight response. Interestingly, this chakra is also linked to a sense of smell.

Muladhara hones one's sense of security, and also chisels basic human potential.

This chakra is associated with the colour red, and is located at the base of the spine in the coccygeal region. It corresponds to the gonads and the adrenal medulla and, at a more general level, the legs, feet, bones and large intestine.

Awakening the Kundalini and Chakra Meditation

Now that we've plotted out the nadis and chakras, we can approach the fascinating subject of kundalini. References to this word are found in tantric manuscripts from the eleventh century, but it is the sixteenth-century text, Yoga Upanishad, that codifies kundalini yoga the way it is known today in the hatha yoga tradition. It describes kundalini as lying 'coiled' in the astral body in the muladhara chakra. Through pranayama, the nadis—particularly ida and pingala—get purified, the chakras are activated and kundalini energy gets awakened.

When awakened, the kundalini is said to uncoil, rise up—chakra to chakra along the central nadi, sushumna—until it reaches the sahasrara chakra at the top of the head. Even as the kundalini progresses through sushumna, one experiences varied levels of awakening and a range of mystical experiences. When it finally reaches the sahasrara chakra, one is said to have reached a place of perfect detachment from both the body and mind; the soul is free.

Kundalini energy in tantrism is also explained in these terms: Shiva resides in the sahasrara chakra and Shakti in muladhara. When they unite in sahasrara, knowledge, the knower and the object of knowledge become one. All desire evaporates because one realizes unequivocally that everything one has ever yearned for is already within. In this state of absolute consciousness, there are no polarities and, therefore, there's no dissipating joy, no lingering sorrow—only everlasting bliss, unconditional love, unlimited compassion and total empathy for all living beings.

■

Particularly beneficial at this level is chakra meditation. As we've established, each chakra is connected to the health of certain organs and glands (in close proximity to where it's located). It is also responsible for certain emotional states and mental characteristics.

To heal and balance the body as well as to find psychological and mental balance, you can try opening, healing and balancing the chakras through chakra meditation—which can take many forms.

Bhuta shuddhi, for instance—an ancient chakra meditation technique used in both the yogic and tantric tradition—is particularly useful as a first step to awaken the kundalini or even to feel poised and stable. The aim here is to progressively move one's awareness through the 'wheels of spinning energy'; intense focus is accompanied by alertness to the nature of each chakra. While practising bhuta shuddhi, the five elements (bhutas) of earth, air, fire, water and ether—which, if you recall, work in conjunction with the lower five chakras—are balanced or purified (shuddhi), and de-blocked, so energy can flow efficiently. (Since the sixth and the seventh chakras, ajna and sahasrara, are associated with the mind and consciousness respectively, they are beyond the scope of the five elements.) As part of the meditation process, the five elements can be purified by reciting bija (seed) mantras (or mystic sounds; more about these later) associated with specific chakras.

This meditation technique is presented below:

To begin with, it helps to perform some stretches or asanas (including partner yoga poses), followed by a short period of relaxation, in order to quieten the mind and prepare it for the sharp focus chakra meditation asks for.

Once this is done, sit in a comfortable, cross-legged position, with your spine straight, shoulders relaxed and eyes gently closed. Take a few full, yogic breaths and progressively focus your attention on the following:

1. Muladhara chakra: Mentally observe the perineum, the flat space between the anus and the genital area. Take your time to get accustomed to focusing on the area, then repeat the mantra 'Lam' (associated with this chakra), at whatever speed comes naturally to you at that moment, and continue to attend to the space assigned to the muladhara chakra. Also, visualize the image of and the concepts associated with the earth, or solidity. Do not get scared if colours and sounds naturally pervade the inner fields of the mind, as this can sometimes happen during meditation.

2. Svadhishthana chakra: Allow your attention to move upwards, and naturally find the location of the second chakra. The actual chakra is at the back of the body, at the level of the sacrum, along the sushumna nadi. However, practitioners usually tend to 'experience' it in the front. Once you've managed to concentrate on this area, start repeating the mantra 'Vam' at whatever speed comes naturally, and continue to focus on the space assigned to the svadhishthana chakra. Picture water and associate it with other forms of fluidity, whether linked to the physical world, or to energy or to emotional or mental qualities. Colours or sounds may manifest themselves—but this is natural. If they don't, don't worry.

3. Manipura chakra: Slowly shift your awareness to the third chakra, at the navel centre, also along the sushumna nadi. Repeat the mantra 'Ram'. Mentally engage with the element of fire and its many variations. Allow colours and sounds to come and go.

4. Anahata chakra: Observe how your awareness moves upwards to the fourth chakra, occupying the space between the breasts, in the territory of the heart. Mentally chant the mantra 'Yam' at a speed that feels natural. Focus on the element of air, its many forms, and notice how that works in conjunction with the mantra. Colours and sounds may come and go.

5. Vishuddha chakra: Draw your attention to the fifth chakra, and the space around the throat. Repeat mentally the mantra 'Ham' and sense the emergence of ether or space (which gives birth to air, fire, water and earth) in your inner self. Keep breathing and remain focused, even while noticing subtle feelings that might (or might not) arise from the experience, or the colours or sounds that emerge or dissipate.

6. Ajna chakra: Slowly and mindfully move your awareness upwards to the space between the eyebrows. Chant the mantra 'Om'. Contemplate the fact that, although the mind has no element associated with it, it allows us to perceive all five 'bhutas'. After all, the mind is the recipient of information coming from the ear, skin, eyes, mouth and nose—whether this is in the form of sensations from the physical world or as memories and past experiences that make up our inner world. Let images and impressions come and go, as you continue focusing on the vibrations of the universal sound 'Om'.

7. Sahasrara chakra: Finally, focus on the crown chakra, which is beyond the scope of any element or cognitive sense and has no active means of expression. It is the source from which the mind emerges and is the doorway to pure consciousness itself. The 'mantra' this time is absolute silence, like the pause between each syllable of 'Om'. Your awareness now rests in pure stillness.

After reaching this point, start the descent backwards within sushumna and into your body and the world: bring your attention again to the ajna chakra and mentally repeat the sound 'Om' for a few seconds or even a minute.

Ever mindful, continue going backwards to the vishuddha chakra, recollecting the mantra 'Ham'; from here, slowly and with awareness, focus your attention on the anahata chakra and repeat the mantra 'Yam'. While remaining attentive, continue going further backwards to the manipura chakra and chant the mantra 'Ram'. Now, shift your attention to the svadhishthana chakra and its mantra 'Vam', and finally, return with complete awareness to where you started—in the muladhara chakra—and allow the mantra 'Lam' to permeate your being.

Ideally, you should spend thirty to forty minutes on chakra meditation, allowing three to four minutes for each chakra in the first half of the meditation sequence and about thirty seconds to a minute each in the second half. You might find the process of meditating very short or incredibly long, depending on how familiar you are with the technique and also based on the time of day, your mood, health conditions and so on. In essence, you can meditate for as long as you find it comfortable.

At first, you may find practising the bhuta shuddhi form of chakra meditation a bit confusing—after all, you have to remain alert to a range of mantras, chakra locations and so on. However, give yourself time, remain alert and gradually try and memorize the mantras, the chakras and their interconnection.

After completing bhuta shuddhi, you can meditate for a little while longer. Or else, you can simply enjoy a round of deep breathing, up and down the sushumna channel, mentally repeating the mantra 'Om' or better yet, 'So-hum'—with 'So' going up to the crown and 'hum' going down to the base of the spine.

What is ॐ (Om)?

The syllable Om/Aum serves as a mantra. 'Om', according to Hindu mythology, is known as the 'pranava mantra', the source of all mantras—the original sound of the universe. This school of philosophy believes that before the creation of the universe, there was only one reality, Brahman, and His first manifestation was expressed through the syllable 'Om'.

■

Why have we delved into the complex world of nadis, chakras and kundalini in this book, and specifically vis-à-vis couple's yoga? It is because the proper regulation of prana through the nadis and the chakras can deepen the synchronization between partners. In other words, any form of harmonization begins with the synchronization of the breath.

MANOMAYA KOSHA AND COUPLE'S YOGA

This layer of being is subtler than the preceding two. However, whatever has been practised vis-à-vis the former koshas will show up at the level of the manomaya kosha. In other words, while you may engage with asanas, pranayama or meditation for physical benefits, you will eventually sense the value of yoga beyond the bodily plane—you feel calmer, less fearful; more upbeat—and this is when the manomaya kosha gets activated.

Now let's consider this kosha in the context of couple's yoga. Again, we must return to the example of two buildings with five storeys (representing the two practitioners), with each floor across structures connected by a bridge. In the manomaya kosha you are on the third floor—the floor of the mind and the subconscious, as well as the senses. The bridge between your partner and you is still understated—in that, it hasn't been intellectualized yet; but now is when you start perceiving a connection and becoming aware of it. Consequently, at this stage, your association with the partner starts to grow even deeper; trust gets built; and both of you reach a place of relatively greater comfort in the relationship.

The virtues associated with the manomaya kosha can be honed by couples by performing kriyas or yogic cleansing techniques as part of partner yoga.

Kriyas

Kriyas are yogic cleansing techniques that tap into your body's 'defence mechanism' of removing all waste—especially that which can affect your health. At a literal level, if there's an episode of food poisoning, your stomach writhes in pain, you experience nausea and retch, which, in turn, helps your digestion get back to normal. By expelling a poisonous substance, the body has instinctively protected itself.

Kriyas follow this principle, and can and should be practised along with asanas and breathing exercises; if executed properly and regularly, they help you to become intimately acquainted with your body's internal processes—beyond merely being aware of the muscles, bones and joints—so, you're conscious of your breathing, blood chemistry, internal organs and subtle energies. This kind of mindfulness helps you reach out to another person more holistically. Kriyas, consequently, stimulate a couple's responsiveness to the manomaya kosha while practising partner yoga.

The yoga text, Hatha Yoga Pradipika, describes six main kriyas (shat kriyas). Initially prescribed for those who come with phlegmatic dispositions, today, these kriyas are found to benefit anyone who is exposed to air that is polluted, food that is heavily processed or industrialized, and water that is often contaminated. The six main kriyas follow.

Neti: Nasal Cleansing

Nasal cleansing is performed with the help of a 'neti pot' in which lukewarm water is mixed with a pinch of salt. The beak of the pot is inserted into one nostril and water is poured in, while keeping the head tilted diagonally, 45 degrees away from the pot. The water naturally flows into the nasal passage and comes out of the other nostril. Now, you can raise your head and blow out excess water from your nostril and then start with the other side.

Nauli: Abdominal Churning

Standing and bending forward slightly, exhale and then bring your navel and intestines 'upwards', so that the abdomen is high in the thoracic cavity and resting against the back of the body. Without inhaling, this position should be held as long as possible. Now, contract the right side and then the left side of the abdomen.

Dhauti: Upper Digestive Track Cleansing

This comprises a set of techniques to cleanse the upper digestive tract:

a) Plavini: This entails filling the stomach with air, then releasing it along with the gases in the belly.

b) Kunjal: After drinking four to eight glasses of lukewarm water on an empty stomach, force yourself to vomit by pressing the stomach with one hand and inserting the finger of the other hand towards the back of the throat.

c) Agni sara: After exhaling, bring the navel and the intestines up; without inhaling, relax the abdominal muscles and draw them in again, all in rapid succession. Repeat the pumping.

d) Vastra dhauti: Insert a fine piece of gauze previously dipped in salt-water into the mouth. Slowly chew the gauze, and swallow it little by little, leaving only a small portion outside the mouth. Allow the piece of gauze to remain in contact with the stomach for a few minutes and then draw it out very slowly.

Basti: Colon Cleansing

As the title indicates, this cleanses the colon. As a part of enema therapy, you create a vacuum in the intestines and allow water to be drawn into the lower colon.

Kapalabhati: Cleansing of the Lungs

While this is a kriya, it is usually practised along with pranayama.

Kapalabhati entails contracting the abdominal muscles quickly. To begin with, after a round of deep inhalation, air is forcefully pushed out of the lungs—causing the diaphragm to move up. This is followed by a round of passive inhalation, which makes the abdominal muscles relax and the diaphragm descend. The fast pumping has to be repeated quickly, alternating forceful exhalation with passive inhalation.

Start by pumping twenty to thirty times, and repeat this for three cycles. Immediately suspend the practice if you start feeling dizzy, as you do not want to run the risk of hyperventilating.

Kapalabhati helps purify nasal passages, bronchial tubes and lungs; a significant amount of carbon dioxide is eliminated and oxygen intake increases. Moreover, the constant and rapid movement of the diaphragm stimulates and massages the internal organs, especially the stomach, the pancreas and the liver. Given how rigorously it cleanses the system, this technique literally means 'shining skull' because it makes the practitioner's face glow with good health.

Tratak: Steady Gazing and the Cleansing of the Eyes

Tratak entails steadily gazing, without blinking, at a particular point or object—the flame of a candle, the tip of your nose or even the space between the eyebrows by turning half-closed eyes towards the ajna chakra. This stimulates the nerve centres and the eye muscles, besides enhancing your concentration.

VIJANAMAYA KOSHA AND COUPLE'S YOGA

This kosha, as we know, is viewed as the layer of the intellect and wisdom. When you pierce the layer of the vijanamaya kosha during individual practice, you come to realize that materialistic concerns are unimportant in the larger scheme of things. You also get less flustered by problems that may have once had a huge emotional impact on your everyday routine.

If a couple happens to be working on this kosha, both will necessarily be practising mantras, asanas, pranayama, kriyas and tantric meditation at an advanced level. At this stage, each develops an understanding of herself/himself, and also her/his partner, in terms of how much each body can do, and what can be expected.

Moreover, the partners' subconscious recognition of a connection (realized while engaging with the manomaya kosha) now becomes wholly conscious; there is an acute awareness of the relationship, a deep acceptance of the other and an ethos of respect and comfort. This is the layer that allows harmony to define an association, as also warmth—not only is there physical attraction, but there is also an element of fascination about the partner's personality, thoughts and way of being.

To return to an earlier metaphor, at this layer, the bridge that establishes the connection between the two buildings/partners is composed of the intellect and the discerning capabilities of each partner's mind.

But how is this bridge to be sustained? At this point, meditation becomes the answer.

Meditation

A powerful tool to develop the connection between two partners in the vijanamaya kosha is meditation.

It is said that when the surface of a lake is still, you can clearly see what lies beneath. But if the lake is agitated, or if waves disturb the sand and debris at the bottom, it is impossible to spot anything at all. The mind is like the lake. If calm, you can glean reality; if agitated, it's impossible to look beyond the whirling of thoughts.

With regular meditation, therefore, the mind is tamed and concentration improves. Trivial problems, worries and misunderstandings recede; the differences between couples dissolve; and mutual understanding is enhanced. Lovers now stand to engage more intensely with the vijanamaya kosha.

ANANDAMAYA KOSHA AND COUPLE'S YOGA

For couples practising partner yoga, the anandamaya kosha is associated with enhanced non-verbal communication, and an overwhelming sense of bliss—suffusing the relationship and pervading the self. Now, the ultimate goal of yoga—to 'join', to establish a union, not only at the physical level, but also in the mental, emotional and spiritual planes—is achieved. Two people—after recovering their individual selves, becoming whole—are now one.

To return to an old metaphor, at this layer, the bridge that establishes the connection between the two buildings/partners is composed of joy of the purest kind and absolute awareness. At this point, mantras act as pole stars.

Mantras

At the level of the anandamaya kosha, it is possible for a couple to chant mantras together to reinforce the state of harmony that pervades their relationship, and thus forge an even deeper spiritual union.

A mantra is mystical energy encased in sound. It may be metaphorical or it may come with a literal meaning. But always, it is loaded with spiritual power when elucidated or repeated.

The 'anatomy' of a mantra is fascinating. Each is a combination of sounds derived from the fifty letters of the Sanskrit alphabet. Mantras are (typically) mathematically structured metres, but not necessarily long. They are usually uttered mentally and when repeated (as in japa meditation) calm the mind, intensify concentration and deepen the state of meditation.

If a mantra is chanted with a lover, it facilitates a connection at the highest level—all realized through the anandamaya kosha.

THE PRACTICALITIES OF PARTNER YOGA

TOUCH, TALK, THINK, TRAIN:
A THEORETICAL INITIATION

It is now time to hit the yoga mat and get down to the basics of *practising* partner yoga. Join me, as I take you through the hoops—from basic individual poses, to advanced partner-driven asanas; from postures that suit a pair of beginners, to those that challenge intermediate or advanced practitioners.

Take your time with your collaborator to first experiment with the simple asanas; learn to understand your body in conjunction with your partner's; and only then 'flirt' with the more advanced poses. In fact, it is this thumb-rule that guides the chronology of asanas in this book—they move gradually from stretches to counterbalancing postures.

PARTNER YOGA AND ASANAS

Asanas are important while discussing yoga, but yoga is not only about asanas. However, for the purposes of this segment, let's understand asanas, as they operate within partner yoga. The asanas you perform with another person can be divided into two categories:

Symmetrical asanas: Both partners mirror each other by practising the same pose either individually or by taking each other's help and support. An example would be the 'two pigeons pose' (asana 12 under 'partner yoga') that features later in the book.

Asymmetrical asanas: Here, it may appear as though the partners are practising two different poses. An example would be the 'flying bow pose' (asana 30 under 'partner yoga') that features later in the book.

An important element guiding asanas in partner yoga is the synergy that the two partners create on the yoga mat. Without this, getting into a position and holding it will not be possible. When one partner bends forward as the other arches back, or when one partner pushes while the other pulls, the counterbalancing effect of two opposing forces creates balance and stability. To reap the maximum range of benefits from a posture, as also to maintain an asana, the partners should observe the way in which such synergy operates and how counterbalancing works—both at the physical level (so a sustained stretch, twist or bend is possible, while remaining stable) and at a more subtle level (so each partner senses her/his dependence on the other, and learns that both have equally important roles to play).

Another important cog in the partner yoga wheel is the role assigned to each partner. Inevitably, one partner will receive a stretch or some support, while the other will give/offer it. The roles of the giver and receiver can then be exchanged, so each partner experiences the joys of both duties while executing the same asana.

This helps both to appreciate the importance of not just providing but also accepting—a lesson that is of relevance beyond the yoga mat, too. On the one hand, the giver develops confidence in her/his capacity to sustain another person; to help a partner to reach new levels of a stretch or a twist; and to communicate such that it's possible to adapt to the other's requirements. On the other hand, as the receiver, while s/he may be more passive, s/he finds joy in allowing the partner to attend to matters of stability and balance; letting go; and enjoying the fact that s/he can rely on the other without always being accountable for everything.

The importance of the receiver letting go during a partner

yoga session cannot be emphasized enough. It's imperative for one of the two partners to relax—so the 'receiver's' body remains malleable, can stretch and reach greater depths, and the asana can be successfully executed. Besides, this is valuable while navigating life, too—during everyday interactions, it is sometimes important to allow others to take charge.

PARTNER YOGA WITH AWARENESS

Another word associated with yoga is 'awareness'. Awareness is the ability to perceive (or remain conscious of) events, thoughts, emotions or experienced sensory patterns. When you act without awareness, your position is like that of a sleepwalker who remains unaware of where s/he's going or why. On the other hand, when you act with awareness, you get to focus on the present without getting distracted by thoughts or emotions linked to the past or the future; you get to perceive thoughts before they have acquired emotional power.

The secret to awareness is *watching,* as though you're bearing witness to your own life. The first level of awareness starts with the body—a body that yoga actually reintroduces you to. When a muscle is used for the first time, the brain recognizes it, senses that it may be exploited frequently, so it labels it as an 'unconscious muscle' to conserve energy. When you practise yoga, these 'unconscious muscles' are brought back to awareness, as performing an asana requires you to exert them in ways never attempted before. Gradually, your proprioception gets fine-tuned. This has an impact on your relationship with your partner, when both of you hit the yoga mat, as both of you become alert to where your bodies exist in relation to space.

The second level of awareness is linked to the mind. The mind is known to swing back and forth. Yoga tames it; as Patanjali says: '*Yogaha chitta vritti nirodaha*' ('Yoga is the restraint of thought'). When your mind is aware, you connect with your surroundings, including the people around you. This has an immediate, positive impact during partner yoga sessions.

The third level of awareness is when the mind—that was tamed at the second level—is entirely still. This means, you stop reacting adversely to situations or to what people say, but respond with calm, pondering over your choice of words and tone, no matter how stressful a situation may be. This ensures that you move towards a place of harmony with your yoga partner.

How does all this translate on the yoga mat during a partner yoga session? To begin with, make it a point to observe how your body stretches, bends, curves, and how your synergy with your collaborator supports you, while at the same time allowing you to sink still deeper into the asana. To make mental notes, take it slowly while practising poses.

To increase awareness, avoid making your practice session a mechanical repetition of postures. Rather, try to really understand and observe what your partner and you are doing in each posture—from the moment you enter a pose to the moment you release it—and try to mix and match.

Finally, calm the mind, so you reach the pinnacle of awareness. Some asanas, more than others, allow you to practically experience what awareness is—among these are balancing poses, as they make you focus on the way you distribute your weight to maintain your balance.

Consider, for instance, vrikshasana, described later in the book (asana 24 of 'the preparatory series'). As you get into the pose, by following the instructions listed under 'getting into the asana', remain alert to your palms pressing into each other very gently, and make note of the part of your body that grants you strength to maintain your balance.

There are other aspects to be observed, too:

► The way in which the body's weight is divided between the two feet.

▶ The way in which the body's weight shifts from one foot to the other.

▶ The way in which the arch of the foot gets a comfortable hold on the inside of the thigh.

▶ The way in which the palms press into each other, giving one a 'grip' over the asana.

▶ How you can actually lengthen the spine by simply lifting the torso upwards.

▶ How ensuring that the chin is gently lifted allows the breath to flow effortlessly.

▶ How looking at a point which is slightly higher than eye level helps you hold the asana with greater stability and balance; also, notice how focusing on a point in front of you gives you a better view of where your body is with respect to your surroundings (for example: how far the wall and/or your partner is from you).

Finally, observe your breath. Despite the fact that there are so many details to take care of, you cannot ignore this aspect. The asana is complete only when you can comfortably hold your breath for some time—*sukham sthitharam asanam*.

PARTNER YOGA AND PROPRIOCEPTION

A key element related to touch, vital to a yoga session, is proprioception—the ability of the central nervous system to communicate with and coordinate various parts of the body (explained at greater length in the first section). Here is a simple exercise to experience proprioception as part of a partner yoga session:

1. Stand in front of the mirror just behind your partner.
2. Tell your partner to keep the eyes closed and avoid looking into the mirror.
3. Hold the right arm of your partner (the arm should remain

relaxed) and move it up and down.
4. Tell your partner to move her/his left arm in exactly the same way that you are moving her/his right arm.
5. Move your partner's right arm to the shoulder level and see if s/he manages to bring the left arm to the same level.

Variations: You can choose to bend your partner's right arm and lower it. You can also follow the sequence listed above by letting your partner lie on the back; further, you could guide her/his right leg to move at random angles in a particular order.

Since your partner cannot see the way in which her/his right arm is being moved, but can only internally 'sense' where the arm is in relation to space, this becomes a fun exercise for both of you!

■

While practising partner yoga, you often have to hold your partner—grip her/his ankles, feet or hands—without looking at her/his body. This is possible because of the sense of proprioception every individual is endowed with.

One can see proprioception at work while practising (for instance) the 'flying bow pose' (asana 30 under 'partner yoga'). Here the partner above simply leans back, places her/his back in correspondence with the feet of the partner lying down below. The partner below holds her/his legs at a 90-degree angle, and holds the shoulders of the partner above so that with such support the partner above can arch the back. In order to maintain balance, the partner above grabs her/his own ankles so that the 'bow' is compact around the legs of the partner below.

What's interesting is that when the partner above reaches out to grab the ankles, s/he is already in an inverted position, and unable to see that area of the body. Now, if the partner above has a good sense of proprioception, s/he will be able to find the ankles easily without having to struggle or grope—in other words, without losing balance. It will be as though the hands have eyes.

If your partner's or your own sense of proprioception is not very good, do not worry! The beauty of partner yoga is that both of you are there to help each other. During practice sessions and even while holding an asana, you can communicate with each other. In the case of the 'flying bow pose', the partner below can gently guide the hands of the partner above towards the ankles, if necessary, to maintain one another's sense of equilibrium.

PARTNER YOGA AND BREATHING

During a partner yoga session, it is crucial that you pay special attention to your breath, as also your partner's, as this will enhance stability, induce awareness and calm the mind.

But what has breath control got to do with serenity of thought? A lot. While searching for methods to calm the mind, pioneering yogis discovered that if they could stabilize their breath, they could restrain mental vacillation. Over the centuries, they developed this discovery into a practice called pranayama—described earlier in the book.

So, let's consider the way we breathe. Normally, when we're not paying attention to how we inhale or exhale, the process can be quite ad hoc—with the intake of air fluctuating depending on our mood, thoughts, the temperature or our diet. Besides, most people use only a fraction of their lung capacity. This is evident in the fact that there are actually *three* types of breathing, and not all of them are ideal:

1. Clavicular breathing, which is the most shallow: The shoulders and collarbone rise while the abdomen contracts during each inhalation. A lot of effort is made, but only a minimal amount of air is retrieved.
2. Thoracic breathing: The rib muscles expand the ribcage, the chest rises, while the abdomen contracts during each

inhalation. Though deeper than clavicular breathing, these gulps of air are also incomplete.

3. Deep abdominal breathing: This brings air to the lowest and largest part of the lungs. The abdomen expands outward as one inhales and contracts as one exhales. Breathing is slow and deep, and the diaphragm is well utilized.

A full yogic breath combines all three types of breathing—beginning with a deep breath, and continuing the process of inhalation through the intercostal and clavicular areas. As one respires in slowly, the abdomen expands, then the ribcage and finally, the upper portion of the lungs. One breathes out in the same manner, letting the abdomen cave in.

At the very least, breathing properly will enhance the benefit of combined asanas, as the cells in the body will be provided with a more abundant supply of oxygen—which, in turn, will grant the muscles the nutrients they crave and reduce fatigue and strain. Equally, proper breathing will calm and sharpen the mind, and enhance awareness, which will grant immense stability to the postures associated with partner yoga.

PARTNER YOGA AND COMMUNICATION

Partner yoga sessions (and indeed, all healthy relationships) are governed by communication. In order to create an atmosphere that is secure, interacting efficiently is vital.

To achieve this end, you need to be a good listener; you need to pay attention to your partner's words and feelings, and directly or indirectly send positive messages that convey your concern. Equally, you need to be a good conversationalist; you need to express your thoughts and feelings without reserve through a careful choice of words, tones, facial expressions and gestures, instead of expecting a partner to read your mind, or getting overwhelmed by a crisis of confidence and the fear that you could cause offence.

As complicated as this sounds theoretically, it is actually fun to practise in the relaxing and playful environment that partner yoga creates. Breathing together, laughing as one when poses become tricky, or correcting an alignment through eye contact are all ways and means of conveying messages. In fact, as you lay aside differences, work in harmony to achieve a common goal and practise communication on the yoga mat, all your relationships in the outside world come to be defined by a similar kind of ease.

So, let's list the ways in which two partners communicate during a partner yoga session:

Words

The most direct means of conveying a message is through words. The golden rule is to say what you need to in the clearest possible manner and encourage the partner by using affirmative expressions. It is particularly important that you let your partner verbally know that s/he is safe and is being supported by you while you are practising an advanced asana.

Touch

Touch, as we've established, is a form of communication. The type of touch, the pressure you apply and the ways in which you reach out for your partner's body communicate your capacity to keep your partner secure. Your touch can also guide your partner with the ways in which s/he is to move her/his body to increase comfort, get a better grip or even improve the overall balance. Moreover, many partner yoga asanas bring together the bodies of the two practitioners in such a way that they allow one or the other to offer a gentle massage.

Eye Contact and Facial Expressions

Looking into the eyes of your partner, whenever your asana permits it, allows both to practise in tandem. Along with this, your facial expressions and those of your partner can communicate a lot. Even if your partner does not admit it verbally, any kind of discomfort on her/his face indicates that the grip/position/stretch needs to be adapted.

An example of such communication between partners can be best observed during the 'riding the boat pose' (asana 6 under 'partner yoga'). This asana, more than others, demands teamwork as well as the coordination of the core muscles of both partners. If you are performing this pose—which looks deceptively simple—for the first time, you need to have a talk with your partner before you begin, so you know how you are to maintain your balance. Once you have managed to get into the asana, you need to continue communicating to ensure that your partner is comfortable with the pressure of the pull/push, and that neither of you is straining the other beyond permissible limits. Throughout, you'll maintain honest eye contact—this is inevitable since both of you sit face-to-face; any kind of discomfort will be immediately discernible.

Why is Safety Vital to Partner Yoga?

Performing asanas with a partner can be fun. The push-and-pull and the counterbalance offered by another body allow you to maintain balance effortlessly, and explore positions in ways you never thought possible during individual practice sessions.

However, partner yoga is only fun when it's safe, done under an expert's guidance and after medical permission. Make sure you first practise the sequences for beginners until you master them. As partner yoga practice advances and both you and your partner gain confidence while holding and lifting each other, you can move to the more advanced poses.

TELL ME WHY:
PARTNER YOGA FAQS

Some of the questions practitioners ask, before commencing a session of partner yoga, include:

HOW OFTEN?

If you are new to this form of yoga, aim for at least one partner yoga practice session a week besides your regular class (assuming you attend a class), and gradually increase the frequency. As you sense the impact of yoga on your body and mind, you will find yourself instinctively stepping onto your yoga mat; this is a sign that yoga is becoming integral to your existence.

WHERE?

Spend some time choosing the best place for partner yoga. While it can be practised virtually anywhere—from a park to your living room—make sure you have enough space to move forward, backwards, left and right without running into or hitting anything. Choose a place with abundant natural light to increase the benefits you derive from yoga. All in all, the place where you practise partner yoga should be comfortable and inspire a sense of well-being.

WHEN?

It is often said that practising yoga at the same time and in the same place is most beneficial. As your mind and body associate set hours and a specific environment with a certain ethic, you find yourself gaining in resolve and motivation.

Having said that, there are no rigid rules about when to practise yoga and whether to follow a routine. If there is one directive, it's this: choose a time when there will be no interruption or distraction, and when you're free of professional or personal commitments. Only then can you sink into the present moment and get absorbed by your yoga practice session.

Another important suggestion to bear in mind: practise yoga on an empty stomach; ensure that there is a gap of two to four hours between your meal and your yoga practice.

WHICH ASANA?

Choose sequences that work for you *now*. The asana bank provided in this book will help you select the most beneficial series based on whether you are a beginner, an intermediate student or very flexible and/or an advanced practitioner. While a bit of challenge is always good, play it safe, especially if you and/or your partner are still relatively new to the concept of yoga.

IN WHAT WAY?

Go slowly, especially in the beginning, and listen to your body. It knows what it can do. If it says 'stop', stop. Don't push it. Yoga is not a competitive sport. If you force your body to go beyond permissible limits, you probably won't enjoy the yoga session, and worse, might end up hurting yourself. Whenever possible, practise yoga under the supervision of a teacher. Most of all, be consistent with yoga sessions: the more you practise yoga, the better you'll understand your body.

Avoid tight outfits and wear comfortable clothes that grant freedom of movement, and leave the abdominal area and ribcage free to expand. Lay down a sticky yoga mat and have an extra mat or a cushion handy to pad your knees or support your back or neck if needed.

THE PREPARATORY SERIES

Partner yoga is a great way to grow together. But it is important for both entities to first hone individual poses to gain in flexibility, strength and stamina. To this end, a preparatory series of asanas is presented before the partner yoga compendium. While performing these asanas, a partner's help is always useful—hence, each preparatory pose comes with a segment suggesting how a companion can help.

ASANA 1: BHARADVAJASANA (BHARADVAJ'S TWIST)

METHOD

Getting into the Asana

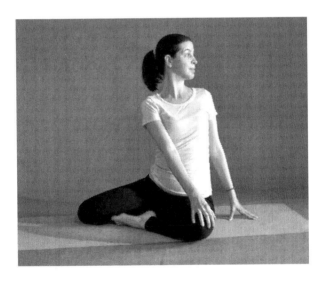

1. Sit on the mat with your legs stretched in front of you. Shift your body weight to your left hip, and bend your legs towards the right. Place your feet on the mat near your right hip.
2. Take in a long, deep breath and lift yourself from the base of the spine to increase the entire length of the torso. Then, release your breath and twist your torso to the left, keeping

the right buttock on (or very close to) the mat. Lengthen your tailbone towards the mat so the lower back remains long.

3. Make a fist out of your right hand and tuck it into the outer side of your left knee. Press your left palm into the mat just next to the tailbone with your arm parallel to the spine. Roll your left shoulder blade back, keeping your chin in line with your shoulder behind. Look as far as you can. Continue to twist your spine with every release of breath.

Maintaining the Asana

1. Secure the body's weight on the palm behind. Maintain the whole length of the spine, by continuing to push into the mat and lifting the crown of the head still higher. The inhalations help you make the spine taller and the exhalations help the spine twist further.

2. Hold the asana for eight to ten long, deep breaths, then release with an exhalation; return to the starting position. Repeat the posture with the other side.

Coming out of the Asana

Stretch the legs out in front of you and relax.

MODIFICATIONS

If sitting on the floor/mat is a challenge, you can use a chair to perform a similar spinal twist. Sit with the back of the chair to your left. Keep your feet firmly on the floor/mat right under your knees. Look towards your left and hold the corners of the back-support of the chair. Keeping the elbows at shoulder level, release your breath and twist the upper body using the strength of your arms as you look over the left shoulder. Keep twisting with every release of breath. Keep the inhalations long, and complete every exhalation. Repeat with the other side.

OBSERVATIONS

Observe the movement of the torso on account of the long inhalations and complete exhalations. Focus on the movement of the navel as well, as it moves in and out. Engaging the abdominal muscles can help extend the duration of the exhalations and promote slow and effortless breathing.

ADVICE FOR THE PRACTITIONER

Bharadvajasana helps twist the spine. You can comfortably hold the position while breathing in and out softly. Closing the eyes will make you feel calm and more acutely aware of the movement of breath.

Avoid straining the shoulder, arm or the side of the neck while trying to achieve a deep spinal twist. Take your time while settling into the asana. Think of this as a preparatory pose for all spinal twists under the partner yoga section.

PARTNERING

A partner can help you sink deeper into the spinal twist. Ask the partner to stand on her/his knees right behind you as you perform the asana. Twist on your own; let the partner place her/his hand on your shoulders and help you twist further.

VARIATIONS

Once you're comfortable in Bharadvajasana, you could attempt the following variation.

Bharadvajasana II: Sit on the mat in a cross-legged position. Place your left palm behind, next to the tailbone, in such a way that your arm stays parallel to the spine. Extend your right arm out, make a fist out of the palm and tuck it into the outer side of the left knee. Press against the left knee to sink deeper into the twist and roll your left shoulder back. Maintain the chin in line with the shoulder behind; look as far as you can over the left shoulder. Keep pushing the left palm down into the mat to lengthen the spine. Continue breathing in and out.

BENEFITS

Bharadvajasana and its variation help:

- lengthen the spine
- relieve lower backache
- stretch the hips and the shoulders
- massage the abdominal organs
- relieve stress
- improve blood circulation

CONTRAINDICATIONS AND CAUTIONS

This asana should be avoided if you're battling diarrhoea; headaches; high blood pressure; insomnia; and/or low blood pressure.

ASANA 2: PADANGUSTHASANA (FEET-TO-FINGERS FORWARD BEND)

METHOD

Getting into the Asana

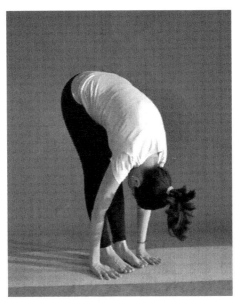

1. Start by standing straight, with your feet parallel to each other and the heels right under the hip girdle. Lift both your arms up, placing them next to your ears. Keeping your legs completely straight, release your breath and bend forward from your hip joint as you push your hips backwards, shifting

the body weight towards your heels. Keep your shoulders and neck relaxed.

2. Grab your toes firmly with your fingers. While exhaling, use the grip of the fingers and the strength of the arms to press your chest towards your thighs. Lift the tailbone up and ensure your body weight remains shifted (towards the heels).

3. Move your elbows away from each other so that the forward bend is induced right from the base of the spine. This will allow the abdomen to go deeper towards the thighs, producing warmth and a comfortable stretch to the hamstrings.

4. This bears repetition: make sure that your head, shoulders and back of the neck remain totally relaxed. Allow your upper body to feel the pull of gravity.

Maintaining the Asana

1. Continue breathing in and out. Every inhalation lifts your body up very gently, and every exhalation creates more space for your body to bend forward, from the base of your spine. Lift your sitting bones as you consciously relax your hamstrings.

2. Hold the final position for five to eight deep breaths.

Coming out of the Asana

1. Relax your toes and let your arm hang down loose.

2. Slowly come up vertebra by vertebra, with the head emerging last.

MODIFICATIONS

If you have very flexible hamstrings, you can press your forehead towards your shins. Focus on folding the body right from the base of your spine, so that the arc deepens; you can let your abdomen touch your thighs.

OBSERVATIONS

Observe how shifting your body weight from your heels to your toes changes the way the hamstrings get stretched. Experience how letting your arms hang loose relaxes the shoulder blades. Pay attention to how it feels when the blood rushes towards your face and the weight of the head pulls the spine down. In this position, exhalations slow down. Lifting the tailbone up and pulling the kneecaps in will also grant a wonderful stretch along the hamstrings.

ADVICE FOR THE PRACTITIONER

Remember that *feeling* the stretch is more important than touching the toes with your hands. If you cannot hold your toes easily while keeping your legs straight, just bend the knees to the extent that feels comfortable, and let your arms hang loose.

PARTNERING

While you're performing the asana, a partner can enhance your awareness of any tension in your muscles by gently touching the back of your neck when you are bending and reminding you to keep your muscles relaxed.

VARIATIONS

Once you're comfortable in padangusthasana, you could attempt the following variation.

Paschimottanasana (forward bend pose): Sit with your legs stretched out in front of you. Get your spine straight, raise your arms up and flex your feet in. Move your arms forward and then down, bending your body from the base of the spine. Grab your toes, pulling them in towards yourself. Slide the heels out to increase the stretch being offered to the hamstrings. Hold the position for a few deep breaths; every exhalation brings you further down, with the forehead towards the knees. While in this posture, you can tuck the chin in towards the chest. To come out of the asana, release your grip on the toes, lift your arms up and then lower your arms down.

BENEFITS

Padangusthasana and its variation help:

- stretch the hamstrings and calves
- strengthen the thighs
- calm the breath
- improve digestion
- improve blood circulation
- relieve stress and anxiety

CONTRAINDICATIONS AND CAUTIONS

This asana should be avoided if you're battling high blood pressure and/or lower back issues.

ASANA 3: NAUKASANA
(FULL BOAT POSE)

METHOD

Getting into the Asana

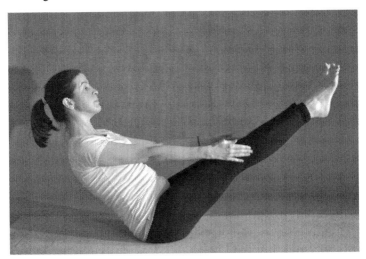

1. Sit on the mat with your legs straight and stretched out in front of you. Hold your spine completely straight. Lift your arms up and stretch them out forward and parallel to your legs. Lift your chin up and lean back using core strength.
2. As you do this, make sure that your back remains totally straight; continue to lift the chest up, away from the chest-bone. Sit on your two sitting bones and your tailbone.

3. Release your breath gently and shift your body weight towards the back while lifting your feet off the mat. Keep your core firm and stable and the arms stretched out parallel to each other and to the floor. Now, slowly straighten your legs and bring your toes to the same level as your eyes and hands.

Maintaining the Asana

1. Continue breathing in and out. Focus on the exhalations and release your breath completely to activate your core muscles.
2. Keep your chin lifted up so that your spine remains straight; avoid curling your spine.
3. Maintain your eyes, hands and toes at the same level. If you feel any kind of pressure on your tailbone, bend your knees, keep the shins parallel to the floor, while ensuring that your body weight remains shifted towards the back; lift your chest up.
4. Remember to keep your arms stretched out and parallel to each other, and to the floor. Spread the shoulder blades away from the spine. If stretching the arms out is not possible, keep your hands on the mat beside your hips, or hold on to the back of your thighs.
5. Hold the pose for four to five long breaths.

Coming out of the Asana

1. Bend your knees and place your feet down on the mat, then come up to a sitting position.
2. Another way of coming out of this asana is by moving your arms over your head. This makes the asana slightly more challenging and fun.

MODIFICATIONS

You can bring your hands close to each other, which shifts your body weight towards the centre of the asana—thus stabilizing the pose and making it easy to hold.

In order to make the abdominal muscles work, you can open the arms to the sides at the shoulder level; this makes the body spread its weight and the core has to keep the body together by providing firmness and stability. At this point, softening the knees can be helpful.

There are two ways of getting into the asana: one option is to advance from a 'lying down position' to naukasana; the other option is to get into the asana from a seated position. Practise both and see what works better for your body type. In both cases, the asana is likely to look exactly the same, but the dynamics and the intensity with which the muscles are activated will vary.

OBSERVATIONS

Observe how the core muscles hold the body together; by moving the arms and legs wide, there will be a shift in the centre of gravity. As you build your core strength, the coordination of the muscles and synchronization of breath will improve.

ADVICE FOR THE PRACTITIONER

Some practitioners may feel that the asana hurts their lower back. This happens because the weight of the legs and the upper body are not well distributed, or because the point of contact with the mat is the lower back or the tailbone. Explore modifications, such as those presented in this segment.

PARTNERING

A partner can sit by your soles and help you hold your feet at the appropriate level by balancing your body's weight against her/his hands. Alternatively, you can have the partner sit next to you, towards your back. You can place her/his hand right between your shoulder blades to offer gentle support while your back remains lifted up.

VARIATIONS

Once you're comfortable in naukasana, you could attempt the following variation.

Ardha navasana (half boat pose): Stretch the arms out to the sides at your shoulder level. Bend your arms and interlock your fingers right behind your head as you curl your spine in and you lower your feet towards the mat. Hold this position, keeping your abdominal muscles active; focus on the exhalations and the movement of your navel.

BENEFITS

Naukasana and its variation help:

- strengthen the upper and lower abdominal muscles
- strengthen the arms and shoulders
- improve breath control
- improve muscle coordination
- massage the internal organs
- improve digestion
- relieve stress

CONTRAINDICATIONS AND CAUTIONS

This asana should be avoided if you're battling asthma; diarrhoea; headaches; heart problems; insomnia; and low blood pressure. Pregnant or menstruating women, too, should avoid this pose.

ASANA 4: BADDHA KONASANA (BOUND ANGLE POSE)

METHOD

Getting into the Asana

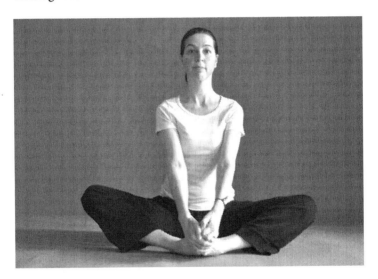

1. Sit on the mat with your legs stretched out in front of you. Release your breath, bend your knees and pull your heels towards your perineum.
2. Lower your knees out to the sides gently, and press the soles of your feet together.
3. Interlock your fingers over your toes and slide your heels as close to your perineum as you comfortably can.

4. Now pull your chest back and hold your spine as straight as you can. Keep your arms straight.

5. Push your abdomen forward and lower your shoulders away from your ears. Keep the chin gently lifted.

Maintaining the Asana

1. Keep the spine totally upright and the chest right on top of the hips.

2. Slow down your respiration and visualize the way your breath moves in and out.

3. Stay in this pose for as long as five to eight long breaths.

Coming out of the Asana

1. Release your grip over your toes. Allow your knees to relax.

2. Stretch your legs out and ease yourself into a comfortable sitting position.

MODIFICATIONS

If your lower back folds easily and a forward bend is effortless, you can stretch your arms out, and lower your body down, so your spine is parallel to the mat. Allow your elbows to be placed gently on the mat, so that all the muscle groups in the upper body can relax.

Later, stretch your arms completely, keeping them parallel to the floor. Using your upper and lower back muscles, pull your torso up and keep your arms in line with the spine. Avoid this modification if you feel any discomfort in your lower back.

Once you are upright, gently place your palms on your knees with the fingers pointing towards your abdomen; keep the elbows bent and pointing outwards.

OBSERVATIONS

Notice how the soles of the feet remain pushed into each other as you slide your heels close to the perineum. Letting your torso lean forward also helps the soles press into each other, besides relaxing the thighs—this makes assuming the asana relatively effortless, and also allows the knees to sink towards the mat. The perineum will then be approximately parallel to the floor and the pelvis in its neutral position. Firm the sacrum and shoulder blades in relation to the back and lengthen the front torso along the top of the sternum.

ADVICE FOR THE PRACTITIONER

Avoid pushing the knees down to the mat. Instead, relax the thighs and let gravity and the weight of the upper body do their job. If your lower back is not very flexible, use a cushion—this helps distribute the body weight properly.

PARTNERING

A partner can assist you with your attempts at lengthening your spine and working on intervertebral spaces. Perform baddha konasana and raise your arms up at 90 degrees, so that they are in line with your spine and perpendicular to the floor. Your partner stands right behind you and places her/his foot behind your lower back, keeping her/his leg parallel to your spine. This allows your spine to remain upright and appear tall. Your partner now holds your arms up and pulls them up slowly, letting your spine grow still taller.

BENEFITS

Baddha konasana helps:

- strengthen the upper and lower back by activating the muscles surrounding the spine
- strengthen the shoulders and deltoid muscles
- stretch the inner thighs, groin and knees

- stimulate the abdominal organs, ovaries, prostate gland, bladder and kidneys
- stimulate the heart and improve blood circulation
- improve inhalation and lung capacity
- destroy diseases and get rid of fatigue (according to traditional texts)
- address sciatica
- address issues that emerge on account of flat feet
- soothe menstrual discomfort
- relieve symptoms of menopause
- ease childbirth if practised until late pregnancy
- address high blood pressure, infertility and asthma
- relieve mild forms of depression, anxiety and fatigue

CONTRAINDICATIONS AND CAUTIONS

This asana should be avoided if you're battling a hip or knee injury, lower back stress and/or a neck injury.

ASANA 5: DHANURASANA (BOW POSE)

METHOD

Getting into the Asana

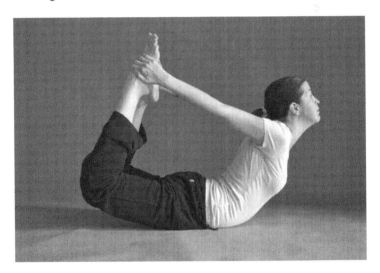

1. Lie down on your belly with your hands next to your body, palms facing up.
2. Gently stretch your arms forward and take a long, deep breath; then lift your legs and arms off the mat.
3. Using your lower back muscles, maintain this position with your chest off the mat.
4. Breathe out slowly and bend your knees, bringing your heels

as close as you can to your buttocks. Reach back with your hands and hold your ankles.

5. Keep your knees narrower than your hips. Now start moving the heels away from the buttocks and let your arms be pulled away with the strength of the thighs.

6. Lift your chin up and draw your shoulder blades towards each other, letting your chest expand. Focus on the inhalations.

7. Push your tailbone down towards the mat, and keep your back muscles relaxed as you continue sending your heels and thighs higher and higher, and away from the hips.

8. Lower your shoulders away from your ears. Look forward by gently lifting your chin.

Maintaining the Asana

1. Keep pushing your heels away from your hips using the strength of your thighs.

2. Focus on inhaling and let your chest expand every time your breath flows into your lungs.

3. Keep your knees wide apart.

4. Stay in this pose for three to five long, deep breaths. Avoid straining your arms. Simply let the strength of the legs pull the arms and deepen the arch in the back. Keep your lower back muscles relaxed too.

Coming out of the Asana

1. Relax the muscles of your thighs and lower back.

2. Lower your feet down to your hips.

3. Lower your forehead down to the mat.

4. Release your ankles and allow your legs to come down.

MODIFICATIONS

If you find it hard to hold both your ankles, try holding your ankles one by one. If the ankles are still out of your grasp, wrap a strap around your feet and grab the strap. You can also try holding your toes.

OBSERVATIONS

This pose is called dhanurasana because of its resemblance to the shape of a bow. So when you are in the asana, visualize yourself arched like one.

Observe the way you breathe. Keeping your breath deep and slow can be a bit challenging as the tummy is pushed towards the mat with the body's weight on it. Allow yourself to make your breath slow but shallow.

Notice how keeping your thighs active makes the arching of the back effortless as the arms are pulled away from the body. You can increase the challenge of dhanurasana by performing the pose by bringing your thighs, calves and inner feet close to each other.

ADVICE FOR THE PRACTITIONER

Keep the neck, shoulders and buttocks relaxed. This allows the back to arch better. Use the strength of the thighs rather than that of the arms. For greater comfort, lay out a thick mat to practise the asana.

PARTNERING

A partner can help you deepen the arch in the back, even while making the asana effortless. Have your partner sit close to your head and place her/his hands on your shoulders. Communicate with your partner and let her/him gently apply pressure in a direction parallel to the floor. This allows you to lift your torso and shift your body weight towards your thighs; your belly is lifted off the mat, you breathe effortlessly and deepen the arch in your lower back. Slowly, your partner will release the pressure, letting your abdomen settle on the mat.

Your partner can also do this by standing behind you, towards your feet. Let her/him grab your ankles and pull them gently in a direction parallel to the floor. This brings about the same effect—lengthening your breath and increasing the intensity of the arch.

BENEFITS

Dhanurasana helps:

- stretch the front of the body, as also the ankles, thighs and groin, abdomen and chest, and the throat
- strengthen the thighs
- stimulate the internal organs in the abdominal region
- improve the flexibility of the spine, shoulders, neck and ankles
- massage the upper back muscles, especially the muscles between the spine and the shoulder blades
- strengthen the back muscles
- open the chest by expanding the ribcage
- improve inhalation
- improve posture and blood circulation

CONTRAINDICATIONS AND CAUTIONS

This asana should be avoided if you're battling high or low blood pressure; migraine; insomnia; a sensitive lower back; and/or a neck injury.

ASANA 6: SETU BANDHASANA (BRIDGE POSE)

METHOD

Getting into the Asana

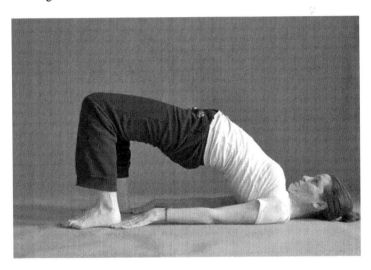

1. Lie on your back on the mat, keeping your neck in line with your spine and your arms totally straight and next to your body, with the palms facing down. Gently bend your knees and place your feet on the mat, parallel to each other and wider than your hips are.
2. Place your feet close to your hips so that your fingers touch your heels.

3. Release your breath and, pressing the soles of your feet and arms firmly into the mat, lift your tailbone upward towards the pubis. Activate your lower back muscles and your buttocks, and then, lift your buttocks off the mat. Keep your thighs and your inner feet parallel.

4. Press into the mat with your hands and interlock your fingers under your pelvis. Squeeze your shoulder blades towards each other. Allow your chest to open and lower it at the same time, keeping your chin close to your chest, and the back of your neck comfortable.

5. Shift your body weight towards your shoulders. Continue to lift your buttocks until your thighs are somewhat parallel to the floor. Keep your knees directly over your heels. Put your lower back muscles and your buttocks to work and squeeze your buttocks in to lift the pubis towards the navel.

6. Keep pressing your hands and your heels into the mat.

Maintaining the Asana

1. Look towards the abdomen and watch the navel rise and fall as your breath goes in and out.

2. Stay in this pose anywhere for five to eight long, deep breaths.

Coming out of the Asana

1. Release the posture with an exhalation, slowly rolling your spine down towards the mat.

2. Stretch your legs out and press your lower back on the mat.

3. Hug your knees to your chest and lift your head up to touch your knees to your forehead.

MODIFICATIONS

If you have difficulty interlocking the fingers behind the back (this could be because your shoulders lack flexibility), allow yourself to grab the ankles and continue pushing your abdomen upwards the same way. You can also grab the border of the mat with both your hands.

OBSERVATIONS

Once in the pose, notice the way your body arches. Observe how squeezing your buttocks and your lower back muscles strengthens the posture and accentuates the arch by lifting the abdomen up by a few inches.

Notice how lifting your heels off the mat allows your body weight to shift towards your shoulders, which gives your interlocked hands more space to push into the mat; this offers an added boost to the arch in the back.

ADVICE FOR THE PRACTITIONER

This is a very important asana and it is used as a counterpose for forward bends like halasana (asana 20 under 'the preparatory series'). Master this pose, if you aim to improve the strength and the flexibility of your lower back. It will work as a building block for many other advanced asanas ahead.

PARTNERING

A partner can help you deepen the asana by standing by your knees (facing you) and pressing your knees with her/his hands—thus applying gentle force in a direction parallel to the floor. Your partner can also help align your neck in line with your spine, which will help you relax the back of your neck.

VARIATIONS

Once you're comfortable in setu bandhasana, you could attempt the following variation.

Suggested variation: Keeping your elbows at the exact same place (as described under 'getting into the asana'), release your fingers and accommodate your arms under your lower back, forming a cup out of your hands. Rest your back on your hands and relax your buttocks and lower back muscles, letting your arms take the weight of your body. The chest expands, and breath flows in effortlessly.

BENEFITS

Setu bandhasana and its variation help:

- stretch the pectorals and the back of the neck
- strengthen the thighs, calves and shoulders
- improve the motion of the shoulder blades
- improve the intake of breath by stretching the walls of the lungs
- stimulate the abdominal organs, the lungs and the thyroid gland
- improve digestion and blood circulation
- relieve the symptoms of menopause
- relieve menstrual discomfort when done with support
- address backaches and headaches
- address asthma, high blood pressure, osteoporosis and sinusitis
- battle insomnia
- calm the brain and elevate the mood
- reduce anxiety and/or fatigue

CONTRAINDICATIONS AND CAUTIONS

This asana should be avoided if you're battling a neck injury (unless you are practising it under the supervision of an experienced teacher).

ASANA 7: USTRASANA
(CAMEL POSE)

METHOD

Getting into the Asana

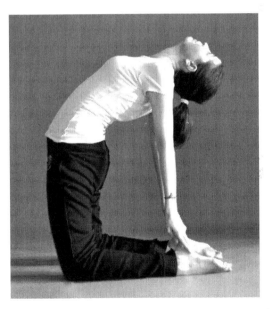

1. Start by standing on your knees and keep them at the same width as your hips, with the thighs perpendicular to the floor. Place your feet so that the space between them is narrower than the space between your shoulder blades, with your toes tucked in and pointing inwards.

2. Exploiting the circular motion afforded by your right shoulder, move your right arm back, bring it down, and hold your right ankle. Move your left arm back the same way and grab your left ankle with your left hand.
3. Rest your hands on your ankles and press them down. Gently shift your body (and the weight it carries) forward towards your knees and squeeze the shoulder blades towards the spine to let the chest expand.
4. Inhale and drop your head back by lifting your chin up.

Maintaining the Asana

1. Keep your body weight on your knees with the hips pointing up.
2. Focus on each intake of breath and expand your chest as the air flows in.
3. Hold this position for three to five breaths.

Coming out of the Asana

1. Shift your body weight to your ankles from the knees by relaxing and pulling your hips back.
2. Gently bring your head back to its normal position by lowering your chin closer to your chest.
3. Draw your arms away from your ankles and stand on your knees.
4. Settle your body into shashankasana (asana 9 under 'the preparatory series') for a few breaths.

MODIFICATIONS

If your back is not flexible at the moment, avoid dropping the head back. Keep the chin close to the chest-bone and look in front. This will ease the pressure on the lower back by shifting the weight of your head towards the front.

Also, you can keep your toes pointed out, letting the top of your feet touch the mat. This will allow you to deepen the arch in the back by pushing the hip girdle forward, bringing the weight of your body towards your knees. You can also place a folded blanket under your knees to avoid any unpleasant pressure to the kneecaps.

OBSERVATIONS

Observe the similarity between the shape of this asana and dhanurasana (asana 5 under 'the preparatory series'). Notice that by bringing the weight of the body to the knees, the back arches gracefully and the shoulder blades squeeze in towards the spine, letting the chest open and expand—thus making the flow of your breath smooth.

ADVICE FOR THE PRACTITIONER

Fold the mat, twice- or thrice-over, under your knees to provide extra cushioning. Remember, keeping the toes tucked in also makes it less challenging for the lower back to arch. You might enjoy enhancing the asana by squeezing your buttocks and your lower back muscles, even as there is a shift in your body weight.

If your back does not arch significantly, you can attempt this asana by involving one arm at a time. So, move your right arm back and grab your right ankle with the toes pointing in. Look over your right shoulder and push the tummy forward. Leave your left arm in front, or place your left hand on the right shoulder. Practising the asana this way introduces a gentle twist. Make sure you repeat this technique with the other side.

PARTNERING

In this pose, a partner can help you improve the posture of your neck and your head. Your partner should stand right behind you as you perform ustrasana. Your partner can place her/his hand behind your head, letting your head lean on it. The other hand of the partner can gently push against your lower back, signalling to the hips that they can move forward and shift the weight towards the knees. Once you gain confidence in the asana and feel comfortable, communicate with your partner and let her/him slowly lower the hand, letting your head tilt back.

VARIATIONS

Once you're comfortable in ustrasana, you could attempt the following variation.

Suggested variation: You can attempt the posture (as described under 'getting into the asana') with the toes pointing out and away from the body, with the top of your feet pressing against the mat. In this variation, the palms will be firmly pressing against the soles of your feet while you arch the back. This allows the practitioner to have an even deeper arch in the back by shifting the body weight towards the knees and pushing the navel forward.

BENEFITS

Ustrasana and its variation help:

- stretch the pectorals and stimulate the neck
- strengthen the lower back muscles, thighs and shoulders
- massage the abdominal organs, lungs and the thyroid gland
- improve the motion of the shoulder blades
- improve posture
- improve inhalation by expanding the ribcage
- battle backaches, headaches
- improve digestion and blood circulation
- relieve menstrual discomfort when done with support
- address asthma, high blood pressure, osteoporosis and sinusitis

- address insomnia
- reduce anxiety and fatigue

CONTRAINDICATIONS AND CAUTIONS

This asana should be avoided if you're battling high or low blood pressure; migraine; a serious lower back injury; a neck injury; and/or vertigo.

ASANA 8: UTKATASANA (CHAIR POSE)

METHOD

Getting into the Asana

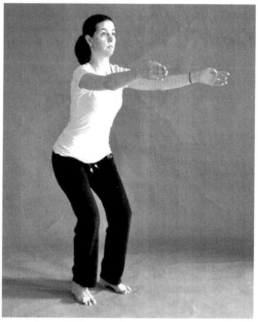

1. Stand tall on the mat with your arms hanging loose by the sides of your body. Inhale and raise your arms parallel to each other and to the floor. Keep the palms facing each other, with the fingers together and pointing out.

2. Release your breath out and bend your knees by lowering your hips, keeping your thighs parallel to each other. Pull your chest back slowly. Hold your head, upper back, hips and ankles in a line with each other.
3. Lift your chin up gently to get your jawline parallel to the floor. Keep your shoulder away from the ears. Tuck your tailbone in, reducing the arch in the lower back so it feels flat and long.

Maintaining the Asana

1. Keep breathing in and out, focusing on every exhalation.
2. The release of breath activates the abdominal muscles; the navel goes in towards the spine, gripping the core to hold the body together.
3. Hold this position for eight to ten long, deep breaths.

Coming out of the Asana

1. Straighten your knees with an intake of breath.
2. Release your breath and now release your arms to your sides.

MODIFICATIONS

You can raise both your arms, keeping them parallel to each other. Hold this position for a few breaths and lower the arms to your shoulder level. Push the shoulders back, letting your chest expand and your breath flow in.

OBSERVATIONS

In utkatasana, watch out for the lower back arching. You can avoid the curling of the spine by tucking the tailbone in. Target keeping the spine straight.

Notice the way each inhalation and exhalation deepens the pose. Watch how the intake of breath is slow and the expulsion of air is complete. Observe how your breath reaches the base of the lungs first, moves towards the upper part of the lungs later, and fills the throat towards the end.

Study the way the navel goes in towards the spine and the abdominal muscles get activated.

Lowering the shoulders down, away from the ears, will save you a lot of energy and make you practise the asana with deeper awareness.

ADVICE FOR THE PRACTITIONER

This pose uses the body as a tool to strengthen the mind. Your body will want to give up after a few breaths. Allow yourself to look beyond the burn in your thighs; convince your body to stay where it is, while remaining aware of the intake and expulsion of breath. Practise tranquillity while performing the asana.

PARTNERING

A partner can help you monitor your breath by reminding you to inhale and exhale long and deep while in the pose. Your partner can also give you feedback, so you can align your head better, and lower your back and your heels.

VARIATIONS

Once you're comfortable in utkatasana, you could attempt the following variation.

Suggested variation: While holding the pose (as described under 'getting into the asana'), lift your heels off the mat, arching your feet. Let your body balance on your toes. You can also extend the arms towards the ceiling, keeping them parallel to each other.

BENEFITS

Utkatasana and its variation help:

- strengthen the ankles, thighs, calves and spine

- stretch the shoulders and the chest
- stimulate the abdominal organs, diaphragm and the heart
- attend to flat feet

CONTRAINDICATIONS AND CAUTIONS

This asana should be avoided if you're battling headaches; insomnia; and/or low blood pressure.

ASANA 9: SHASHANKASANA (CHILD POSE)

METHOD

Getting into the Asana

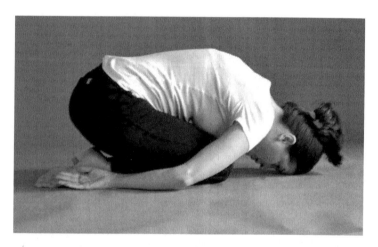

1. Sit on the mat on your knees. Bring your big toes together so that they touch, and now sit on your heels. Keep your knees as wide as your shoulders are.
2. Release your breath and bend your body from the base of the spine; lay your torso between your thighs, and your shoulders between your knees. You can place your forehead on the mat facing down or look to one side—whichever feels comfortable for your neck.

3. Place your hands on the mat alongside your body, keep the palms facing up, and release the front of your shoulders towards the mat. Dropping the front shoulders will allow your shoulder blades to expand.

Maintaining the Asana

1. Relax the back of your neck and the muscles around the shoulders, and let them feel the pull of gravity.
2. Scan your body mentally and experience different levels of relaxation.
3. Stay in this resting position for a couple of minutes.

Coming out of the Asana

1. Bend your arms and place your palms under the shoulders on the mat.
2. Gently press the mat with your hands; simply pull your chest up and bring the spine into an upright position.

MODIFICATIONS

If you have difficulty sitting on your heels in this pose, keep your feet further away from each other. This will let your buttocks sink further down and avoid any kind of weight on the ankles.

OBSERVATIONS

Since your nostrils are very close to the mat in the position, you should be able to listen to the sound of your breath very carefully. Use this opportunity to increase your awareness about the intake and expulsion of air, even while making sure you inhale and exhale effortlessly; avoid any sort of retention. We usually do not breathe consciously and fully into the bottom of the lungs. Shashankasana gives you an opportunity to respire well.

ADVICE FOR THE PRACTITIONER

In shashankasana, your muscles are totally relaxed. Therefore, this position is often used as a counterpose to backward bends and helps cool the body after a challenging asana.

PARTNERING

Have your partner stand to one side of you. S/he should place one hand on your sacrum (fingers pointing towards the tailbone) and the other hand on your mid-back (fingers pointing towards your head). After you exhale smoothly, your partner can—without physically moving her/his hands—push her/his hands in opposite directions to lengthen the spine. Communicate with your partner and help your partner regulate the pressure on your back; ask for more or less force, but remember, have her/him apply more pressure only at the time of the expulsion of air.

VARIATIONS

Once you're comfortable in shashankasana, you could attempt the following variations.

Variation 1: Holding shashankasana (as described under 'getting into the asana'), let your arms stretch out and join the palms together. Keep the palms firmly pushed into each other, bend the arms and bring the hands right behind your neck. Your elbows are resting on the mat, letting your chest sink down towards the mat.

Variation 2: Holding shashankasana (as described under 'getting into the asana'), stretch your arms next to your body and face one side. In other words, let the side of your face touch the mat.

BENEFITS

Shashankasana and its variations help:

- relax the upper back muscles by spreading the shoulder

blades away from each other
- stretch the hips, thighs and ankles gently
- relieve back and neck pain when the head and torso are supported
- promote slow, deep, calm and effortless breathing
- calm the brain and relieve stress and fatigue

Besides, shashankasana helps a practitioner let go, making her/him feel humble, just like a baby.

CONTRAINDICATIONS AND CAUTIONS

This asana should be avoided if you're suffering from diarrhoea and/or a knee injury (in which case, avoid shashankasana unless you are under the supervision of an experienced teacher). Pregnant women should avoid this pose.

ASANA 10: BHUJANGASANA
(COBRA POSE)

METHOD

Getting into the Asana

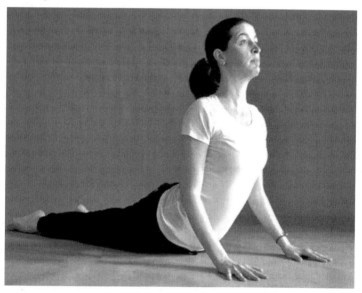

1. Lie down on the mat on your belly. Stretch your legs with the toes pointing out. Place your hands firmly right under your shoulders on the mat. Keep your elbows very close to the ribcage. Your forehead should touch the mat.
2. Take in a long, deep breath, press your palms down into the mat firmly and lift your chest off the mat, reaching a level

where the navel stays in touch with the mat, or goes off the mat by about three inches.

3. Draw your shoulder blades away from your ears. Keep your buttocks relaxed and the big toes in touch with each other.
4. Firm your shoulder blades against your back, lowering them away from the ears. Lift the chin up to maintain a stretch in front of your neck.

Maintaining the Asana

1. Keep your lower back muscles active.
2. Let your triceps take care of the upper body weight.
3. Keep your fingers spread out on the mat.
4. Allow your breath to flow in and out effortlessly.
5. Keep the chin gently lifted.
6. Hold this pose for five to eight long, deep breaths.

Coming out of the Asana

1. Simply bend your arms and lie down with your chest on the mat.
2. Stay in this position and let your back and arms relax.

MODIFICATIONS

If your lower back does not allow you to arch very much, lift your chest to such a level that the back is still comfortable; the lower back should not feel squeezed, and your navel should be in touch with the mat.

If you have a certain amount of flexibility around the armpits, chest and groin, you can move into an even deeper backbend. Walk your hands slightly forward and straighten your elbows, turning your arms outward. Lift the top of the sternum straight towards the ceiling.

OBSERVATIONS

While in this asana, remain conscious of the fact that your lower back muscles and your triceps help you maintain your position. Initially, your body will be tempted to engage your buttocks. Observe how activating your lower back muscles and your triceps allows you to hold the asana without involving your hips. Moreover, the higher you lift your chin away from the navel, the more intense the stretch of your abdominal layer will become with each inhalation.

ADVICE FOR THE PRACTITIONER

Be extra careful with any backward bend. Avoid overdoing it or overworking the muscles around your neck and shoulders. Always pay attention to uniformly dividing the backbend along the spine, instead of putting pressure on one vertebra alone.

Keep your shoulders open and away from the ears to maintain proper blood circulation.

PARTNERING

Your partner can help you make the spine arch better and stabilize the asana by keeping her/his hands on your lower back. Your partner can also sit with her/his legs on either side of your hips and with her/his knees down. As you inhale to lift your torso off the mat, your partner can gently place her/his hands on your shoulders and pull them backwards, so that you can hold the asana with ease.

When you choose to come out of the asana, allow your partner to lower your body down very gently. S/he can also soothe your lower back with a quick massage.

VARIATIONS

Once you're comfortable in bhujangasana, you could attempt the following variation.

Suggested variation: When you are up like a cobra (as described under 'getting into the asana'), look towards the right and align your chin with the right shoulder. Let your upper body twist. Look towards your buttocks over your shoulder. Let a deep intake of breath enter the torso as the body maintains a backbend and a soft twist. Repeat with the other side.

BENEFITS

Bhujangasana and its variation help:

- strengthen the spine
- stretch the chest and lungs, shoulders and abdomen, and open the heart and lungs
- firm the buttocks
- stimulate abdominal organs
- soothe sciatica
- address asthma
- increase body heat, destroy disease and awaken the kundalini (according to traditional texts)
- relieve stress and fatigue

CONTRAINDICATIONS AND CAUTIONS

This asana should be avoided if you're battling a back injury; the carpal tunnel syndrome; and/or headaches. Pregnant women, too, should avoid this pose.

ASANA 11: SAVASANA
(CORPSE POSE)

METHOD

Getting into the Asana

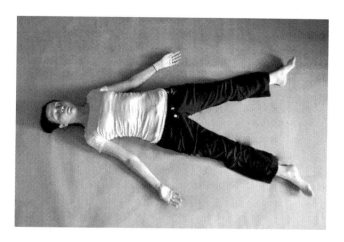

1. Lie down on your back with your arms away from your body, such that your shoulder blades comfortably settle down on the mat.
2. Keep your palms facing up and your arms slightly away from your body.
3. Keep your feet wide apart and drop your toes outwards, letting the ankles relax.
4. Focus on your breath and visualize the navel going up and down with the intake and expulsion of air.

Maintaining the Asana

1. Soften the root of your tongue, the wings of your nose, the channels of your inner ears and the skin on your forehead, especially around the bridge of the nose between the eyebrows.
2. Close your eyes and let them relax; it will feel as though they are sinking to the back of your head.
3. Stay in this pose for five minutes after every half hour of yoga practice.

Coming out of the Asana

1. Exhale and gently turn towards the right.
2. Take two or three breaths.
3. Exhale again, press your hands into the mat and lift your torso, lifting your head slowly after this. The head should always come up last.

MODIFICATIONS

Savasana is usually performed with the legs kept straight. But if you have a deep arch in the lower back, bending your knees and placing your feet close to your hips may be a good idea. This allows the arch of the lower back to reduce and the lumbar region to settle down towards the mat.

It also feels good when this pose is completed with a pillow placed right under the shins. If the back of your head feels uncomfortable, you can slide a thin, firm pillow or a folded blanket right under your head.

OBSERVATIONS

Become aware of the way you breathe. Sense the air entering the nostrils, touching the back of the throat, going down along the spine and settling towards the navel. Perceive the navel moving away from the spine. You'll experience a sense of expansion.

Now feel your breath leave the body. Perceive the way the navel sinks down towards the spine and how the body empties itself out. Imagine the heads of the thigh bones sinking down into the mat. Make note of all the points where the body is in contact with the mat. Allow the muscles to relax and visualize yourself in a beautiful, natural setting.

ADVICE FOR THE PRACTITIONER

This is one of the difficult asanas—and the comment takes everyone by surprise! There is 'nothing much' to be done here. But you must make sure that you do the 'nothing much' properly.

Thoughts will come and go. Do not get bothered with the sounds and the movements around you. You will notice your reflections settling down as your breath relaxes and slows down. You will start loving this asana as you sink deep into it.

PARTNERING

With savasana, it is very useful to have a partner correct your physical alignment. It's a bit tricky to keep your head in line with your spine. Your partner can sit near your head and observe its position relative to your spine and shoulders. It is common for most students' heads to tilt or turn to one side—in which case, your partner should gently cradle your head in her/his hands and draw the base of the skull away from the back of the neck, lengthening the shorter side of the neck, so that both ears are evenly away from the shoulders. Then your partner can lay your head back down on the mat, making sure that the tip of your nose is pointing directly towards the ceiling.

VARIATIONS

Once you're comfortable in savasana, you could attempt the following variation.

Supta baddha konasana (reclining bound angle pose): Once in savasana (as described under 'getting into the asana'), bend your legs and place the soles of your feet together. Drop the knees down and away from each other towards the mat. Allow your legs and your entire body to relax.

BENEFITS

Savasana and its variation help:

- relax and quieten the physical body and pacify the sense organs
- lower blood pressure
- address headaches, fatigue and insomnia
- calm the brain and relieve stress and mild depression

CONTRAINDICATIONS AND CAUTIONS

This asana should be practised with care in case of a back injury or discomfort, or if you are pregnant.

If you're battling a back injury/discomfort: Practise this pose with your knees bent and your feet on the mat, hip-distance apart; either keep the thighs parallel to each other with a strap (taking care not to position the heels too close to the buttocks) or support the bent knees on a bolster.

If you're pregnant, raise your head and chest on a bolster.

ASANA 12: ADHO MUKHA SVANASANA OR PARVATASANA (DOWNWARD-FACING DOG POSE)

METHOD

Getting into the Asana

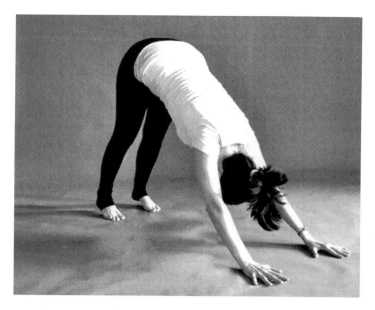

1. Place your knees and palms on the mat. Keep your hands forward in comparison to your shoulders and your knees right under your hips.

2. Point your toes in and grip the mat with them.
3. Spread your fingers wide on the mat and grip the mat well.
4. Firmly push your palms into the mat and slowly and gently lift your knees off the mat.
5. Keep your knees soft and bent, and align your arms and your spine in one line with each other.
6. Keep your neck and head relaxed with your shoulders away from your ears.
7. Pushing your toes into the mat, pull the kneecaps in, push your heels towards the mat and raise your tailbone up towards the ceiling.

Maintaining the Asana

1. Ensure that you keep your neck relaxed once in the asana.
2. Push your heels on the mat one by one to soften the hamstrings.
3. Breathe normally.
4. Hold the position for eight to ten long, deep breaths.

Coming out of the Asana

1. Simply bend your knees on the mat with an exhalation and rest in shashankasana (asana 9 under 'the preparatory series').

MODIFICATIONS

Adho mukha svanasana or parvatasana is one of the poses in the traditional surya namaskar (sun salutation) sequence. It's also an excellent yoga asana in its own right.

To work the outer arms, loop and secure a strap around your arms just above your elbows. Imagine that the strap is tightening inward, pressing the outer arms against the bones. Against this resistance, push the inner shoulder blades outward.

OBSERVATIONS

Feel the stretch being offered to your body. To increase the stretch provided to the back of your legs, lift yourself slightly on the balls of your feet, pulling your heels a half-inch or so away from the mat. Then, lifting actively from the inner heels, draw your groin deep into your pelvis. Finally, from the height of the groin, lengthen the heels back into the mat, moving the outer heels faster than the inner heels.

ADVICE FOR THE PRACTITIONER

This asana might feel uncomfortably challenging in the beginning. Focus on sinking your chest down towards the mat, keeping the spine and the arms in a straight line with each other.

There are many different ways in which adho mukha svanasana or parvatasana can interact with a partner yoga pose—as we'll get to see later in the book. Hence it is important to practise this asana until you start loving it.

PARTNERING

A partner can help you take the hamstring stretch to a whole new level. First get into adho mukha svanasana or parvatasana. Have your partner stand in front of you. Now the partner places her/his hands firmly on your lower back and applies a force parallel to the floor. The aim is to press your heels down towards the mat. Your partner can also bend her/his right knee and place it on your upper back to give a gentle push, which will further align your arms and spine with each other.

VARIATIONS

Once you're comfortable in adho mukha svanasana or parvatasana, you could attempt the following variation.

Suggested variation: To challenge yourself in the pose (as described under 'getting into the asana'), inhale and raise your right leg parallel to your torso, and hold this position for thirty seconds; throughout, keep the hips level and press through the heel. Release with an exhalation and repeat with the left side for the same length of time.

BENEFITS

Adho mukha svanasana and its variation help:

- stretch the shoulders, hamstrings, calves and hands
- strengthen the arms and legs
- energize the body
- improve digestion
- prevent osteoporosis
- relieve the symptoms of menopause
- relieve menstrual discomfort when the head is supported
- relieve headaches, insomnia, back pain and fatigue
- address high blood pressure, asthma, flat feet, sciatica and sinusitis
- calm the brain and relieve stress and mild depression

CONTRAINDICATIONS AND CAUTIONS

This asana should be avoided if you're battling the carpal tunnel syndrome and/or diarrhoea. Pregnant women should skip this pose altogether. If you're a patient of high blood pressure or if you're fighting a headache, support your head on a bolster or a block.

ASANA 13: GARUDASANA
(EAGLE POSE)

METHOD

Getting into the Asana

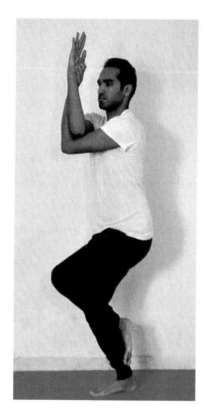

1. Stand tall on the mat. Bend your knees slightly, lift your left foot up and, balancing on your right foot, cross your left thigh over the right.
2. Point your left toes towards the mat, press the foot back, and then tuck the top of the foot behind the lower right calf. Maintain your balance on your right foot.
3. Stretch your arms straight in front of you, parallel to the floor, and spread your shoulder blades wide across the back of your torso. Cross your arms in front of your torso so that the right arm is above the left, then bend your elbows. Place your right elbow on the left arm, and raise your forearms perpendicular to the floor. Join the palms together in the prayer position.
4. Slowly turn the hands so the palms are now facing each other. The thumb of the right hand should pass in front of the little finger of the left hand. Now, press the palms together (as much as is possible for you), lift your elbows up and stretch the fingers towards the ceiling.

Maintaining the Asana

1. Breathe in and out as normal.
2. Lower your hips to keep the top of your right foot tucked behind the calf muscle of your left leg.
3. Keep your elbows at shoulder level and ensure that the expansion of your shoulder blades does not decrease.
4. Hold the pose for eight to ten long, deep breaths. Get back to the starting position. Repeat the asana for the same number of breaths with the arms and legs reversed.

Coming out of the Asana

1. Pull your chest back and unwrap your arms.
2. Raise yourself up and unwrap your legs, and place your feet back on the mat.

MODIFICATIONS

Tucking the foot behind the shin while maintaining your balance on one foot can be a bit tricky. Practise the position with your back leaning against the wall, and sink down along the wall by bending your knees. Keep pushing against the wall and let yourself wrap one leg around the other.

OBSERVATIONS

Observe the body as it is tied into a knot made out of its own limbs, making it very compact and stable. Focus on the flow of the breath and the expansion of the upper back.

ADVICE FOR THE PRACTITIONER

Sinking down into the position helps you wrap one leg around the other. So, lower the hips down by bending one leg, wrap the other leg and tuck the foot in with the shin of the balancing leg. Once the arms are wrapped and the palms are touching each other, pull your chest back to extend the length of the spine and lift the elbows up and away from the knees.

PARTNERING

The partner can stand by your hands and place her/his hands on your lower back, applying force in a direction parallel to the floor. This will help you shift your body weight towards your heels, which in turn, will push the heel of your balancing leg into the mat.

VARIATIONS

Once you're comfortable in garudasana, you could challenge yourself with the following variation.

Suggested variation: Follow the guidelines listed under 'getting into the asana'. Let yourself sink down further with your hips and extend your arms to the sides, maintaining them at shoulder level. Now, lower your chest till it touches your upper thigh and expand your arms as though they are wings. Lift your chin and look forward to get your throat in line with your spine. Switch the position of your legs and repeat.

BENEFITS

Garudasana and its variation help:

- strengthen and stretch the ankles and calves
- stretch the thighs, hips, shoulders and upper back
- address asthma, low backaches and sciatica
- improve a sense of balance
- improve concentration

CONTRAINDICATIONS AND CAUTIONS

Students with knee injuries should avoid this pose, or perform only the leg position described in the 'advice for the practitioner' section.

ASANA 14: SUKHASANA
(EASY POSE)

METHOD

Getting into the Asana

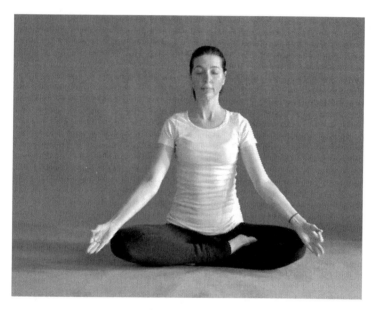

1. Sit on the mat with your legs outstretched and the spine straight. Bend your left leg in such a way that the left foot gets slightly tucked under the right thigh.
2. Now bend your right leg. Slide the left foot under the right shin, letting the left leg rest on top of the right foot.

3. Lift your chest up and align it right above your hips. Place both your hands on top of your knees and lower the shoulders to relax them.

Maintaining the Asana

1. Keep your legs comfortably crossed and the spine upright.
2. Ensure that the hands are resting on top of the knees and your elbows are totally relaxed.
3. The body's weight should be divided between the sides of the feet and the sitting bones.

Coming out of the Asana

1. Stretch your legs and relax.

MODIFICATIONS

If you find sitting in this position uncomfortable, you can use blocks or blankets right under the knees to provide support. This will help you reduce the stretch around the groins and/or the inner thighs. You can also wedge a cushion under your tailbone to keep the spine upright.

OBSERVATIONS

Pay attention to the fact that your elbows start feeling heavy, pulling your shoulders down. Observe how your spine remains straight and your head in line with the spine. Notice the depth of each inhalation, as well as the duration of each exhalation.

ADVICE FOR THE PRACTITIONER

This is a key position for meditation. The aim is to hold sukhasana comfortably for a long duration—entirely possible once the body gains in flexibility. This will allow you to meditate without any physical discomfort.

PARTNERING

The partner can help you align your back with your hips and remind you to focus on your breath. S/he can also urge you to keep your shoulders relaxed in sukhasana.

BENEFITS

Sukhasana helps:

- stretch the knees and ankles
- strengthen the back
- calm the brain

CONTRAINDICATIONS AND CAUTIONS

This asana should be avoided if you're battling a knee injury.

ASANA 15: UTTHITA TRIKONASANA (TRIANGLE POSE)

METHOD

Getting into the Asana

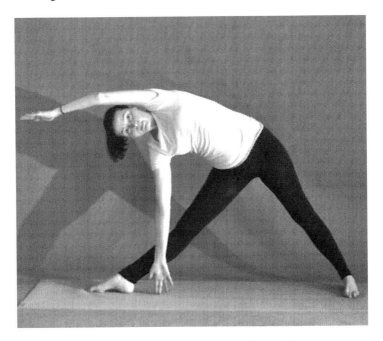

1. Stand straight on the mat. Keep your legs wide apart.
2. Move your arms to shoulder level, parallel to the floor. Align the heels such that they are under the wrists.

3. Point your right foot out in a way that makes it perpendicular to the left foot.
4. Let your left palm face the ceiling and slide your upper body towards where your right foot is pointing.
5. Now lower your right hand onto your right ankle; keep your left arm up, the fingers pointing towards the ceiling.
6. Slowly move your left arm over your head and keep your arm hidden behind your right ear. Keep your fingers pointing out to experience the stretch being offered to the outer side of your torso.

Maintaining the Asana

1. Keep lowering your right hand towards the floor.
2. Push the centre of your body forward, pulling the left shoulder back at the same time.
3. Move your left arm over your head and stay tilted.
4. Continue breathing and, with every release of the breath, see if you can lower your left hand further down.
5. Stay in the asana for fifteen deep breaths.

Coming out of the Asana

1. Stretch your right arm out and ensure that it is parallel to the floor. Start coming up, and inhale as you do so, strongly pressing your left heel into the mat and stretching your left arm towards the ceiling.
2. Pull your chest back, so it is on top of your hips.
3. Lower both your arms down and bring your legs together. Relax.
4. Stay in this pose for thirty seconds to one minute.
5. Repeat the asana for the same number of breaths with the arms and legs reversed.

MODIFICATIONS

If touching the mat with the bottom hand is uncomfortable, simply reach for your ankle or knee, whichever you find convenient to hold. Also, if you feel that your hamstrings are far too tight and holding the legs straight is getting to be uncomfortable, gently soften or bend the knee of the outstretched leg.

OBSERVATIONS

Visualize yourself from above. Ensure that the torso remains right on top of the legs. Sense the pressure of a stretch as it flows from the side of the torso to the hamstrings of the leg inside.

ADVICE FOR THE PRACTITIONER

Usually the chest moves forward in the pose. Press your lower hand on the inside of your ankle and pull your chest back, pushing your abdomen forward.

PARTNERING

This asana is all about proper alignment. It's only if the asana is well-aligned that you will get a most amazing stretch. If not done properly, you might just end up looking like a triangle but not *feeling* like one.

Your partner can help you align yourself properly. Have her/him stand right behind you and help you pull your chest back with her/his left hand on your shoulder. Your partner can also gently press her/his leg against your hip to help you stretch adequately.

VARIATIONS

Once you're comfortable in utthita trikonasana, you could attempt the following variations.

Variation 1: When you are in the position mandated by the asana (as described under 'getting into the asana'), ensure that the left arm points towards the ceiling. Keeping both arms in line, stretch them in opposite directions. Press the back of the right hand against the inside of the right ankle, push the tummy forward and send the left arm further back to keep the body aligned.

Variation 2: Taking off from variation 1, send your left arm back and wrap it around the body, grabbing the right thigh with the left hand, if possible. Roll the left shoulder further out and push your tummy forward. Release the posture and repeat this with the other side.

BENEFITS

Utthita trikonasana and its variations help:

- stretch and strengthen the thighs, knees and ankles
- stretch the hips, groin, hamstrings, calves, shoulders, chest and spine
- stimulate the abdominal organs
- improve digestion
- relieve the symptoms of menopause
- relieve backache, especially through the second trimester of pregnancy
- address anxiety, flat feet, infertility, neck pain, osteoporosis and sciatica
- relieve stress

CONTRAINDICATIONS AND CAUTIONS

This asana should be avoided if you're battling headaches and/or low blood pressure.

If you're a patient of a heart condition, practise against a wall and keep the top arm on the hip.

If you're a patient of high blood pressure, turn the head to gaze down in the final pose.

If you suffer from neck problems, don't turn your head to look upwards; continue looking straight ahead and ensure that both sides of the neck are evenly stretched.

ASANA 16: MATSYASANA (FISH POSE)

METHOD

Getting into the Asana

1. Get into shashankasana (asana 9 under 'the preparatory series'). Keeping your legs in the same position, lift your chest up and slide your feet slightly away from each other, letting your buttocks sink in between your feet.
2. Place both your hands behind you, press your palms on the mat and lean your torso back.
3. Walk your hands away from your feet very slowly and lean further back until your shoulders are right above your wrists, and your arms are perpendicular to the floor and parallel to each other.
4. Bend your arms one by one and place your elbows down on the mat. This will lower your torso backwards.
5. Keeping the chin close to the chest, look towards your knees and arch the back, lifting the navel up.
6. Squeeze your shoulder blades into each other and drop your head back, letting your throat come in line with your spine.
7. Slide your elbows further towards your hips, until the crown of your head touches the mat.

Maintaining the Asana

1. Keep the muscles along the spine active to maintain the supporting arch of the asana. Shift the weight of the upper

body towards the elbows rather than towards the crown of the head.

2. Keep the eyes open.

Coming out of the Asana

1. Grip your ankles with both your hands.
2. Push your elbows firmly into the mat in such a way that the weight of the upper body comes off the crown of the head; you are now able to lower your chin towards the chest, keeping the back off the mat.
3. Grip your ankles still tighter and press the elbows even more firmly into the mat—such that you are able to bring your torso upright. You can press your hands into the mat one by one to help you return to a sitting position.

MODIFICATIONS

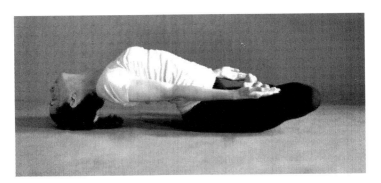

Once you are in the posture (as described under 'getting into the asana') and comfortably placed with the crown of the head on the mat, see if you can lift the elbows off the mat and stretch the arms out, placing the palms on top of your thighs. You can also join the palms together, right in the centre of the chest or send your arms up, over the head, where the hands in a prayer position are visible to you.

The backbend that matsyasana demands can be challenging for beginners. If you find the intricacies of this pose difficult, perform it with a yoga block under the middle of your back.

OBSERVATIONS

While in matsyasana, pay attention to each inhalation and notice the expansion of the chest when you breathe in. Notice the activation of the muscles surrounding the spine and the stretch being offered to the top of your thighs.

ADVICE FOR THE PRACTITIONER

Focus on maintaining the arch of the back as this activates those muscles which provide a cushion to the spine. As the arch deepens, the position becomes even more stable and relatively easy to hold. Since this can be a tricky pose, make sure that you do not hold your breath.

PARTNERING

A partner can make getting into this position effortless. Have your partner stand with her/his feet on either side of your waist. Your partner holds your wrist and pulls your arms towards herself/ himself, and lifts your upper back off the mat. Now you can relax completely without any resistance and lift your chest up, arching your lower back. Lean back with your head, and place the crown of your head on the mat in such a way that your back is off the mat. Your body is in the fish pose, with an incredible backbend and a comfortably positioned neck.

VARIATIONS

There are a few different ways in which to position your legs while in matsyasana. Once you're comfortable in the asana, you could attempt the following variations.

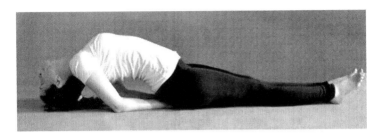

Variation 1: Lie down on your back and keep your legs outstretched. Place your hands behind, on the mat. Bend your arms and place your elbows on the mat, drop your head back, arch your back, lift your chest up, push your elbows further into the mat and slide your hips towards the elbows, letting the crown of your head settle on the mat. This variation is suitable for those practitioners who lack flexibility in the knees and ankles, and find it hard to keep the knees bent with the weight of the body on them.

Variation 2: In this variation, you can cross your legs and get into padmasana (asana 19 under 'the preparatory series')—your left foot is on top of the right thigh and the right foot on top of the left thigh. Both your soles will be facing the ceiling and your heels will be close to your lower abdomen. In this position, place your hands behind, on the mat. Slowly lean back by placing your elbows on the mat. Lift your chest up, arch your back. Slide your hands in towards your hips and place the crown of your head on the mat. To make the position more interesting, stretch the arms out towards your feet and grab your big toes.

BENEFITS

Matysasana and its variations help:

- stretch the deep hip flexors (psoas) and the muscles (intercostals) between the ribs

- stretch and stimulate the muscles of the belly and the front of the neck
- stretch and stimulate the organs of the belly and the throat
- strengthen the muscles of the upper back and the back of the neck
- improve posture
- destroy diseases (according to traditional texts)
- address constipation, respiratory ailments, mild backaches, fatigue, anxiety and menstrual pain

CONTRAINDICATIONS AND CAUTIONS

This asana should be avoided if you're battling high or low blood pressure; migraine; insomnia; a serious lower back injury; and/or a neck injury.

ASANA 17: CHATURANGA DANDASANA (FOUR-LIMBED STAFF POSE)

METHOD

Getting into the Asana

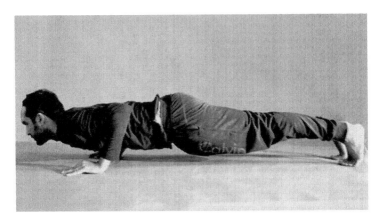

1. Begin with the adho mukha svanasana or parvatasana (asana 12 under 'the preparatory series') and glide the upper body into the push-up position.
2. Press your palms firmly on the mat and align the shoulders, hips, knees and ankles, so that they are in one line with each other.
3. Exhale and slowly lower your torso and legs till they're only a few inches above the mat and parallel to it.

Maintaining the Asana

1. Spread your fingers open as your palm firmly presses into the mat. Keep the core active and the tailbone slightly lifted up.
2. Keep the elbows close to the ribcage and the chin pointed out to ensure that the throat is parallel to the floor. Slow down your respiration.

Coming out of the Asana

1. Press your palms firmly on the mat and raise your body up.
2. Fold your body from the base of the spine and glide into adho mukha svanasana or parvatasana (asana 12 under 'the preparatory series').
3. Gently lower your knees to the mat and lower the hips on the heels, folding the body into shashankasana (asana 9 under 'the preparatory series').
4. Raise your torso and settle into a seated posture.

MODIFICATIONS

Keep the tailbone slightly raised, as this lowers the challenge of holding the body parallel to and just above the mat. You can also place the knees on the mat gently for extra support, but keep your chest off the mat and the arms bent, with your elbows next to the ribcage.

OBSERVATIONS

Notice how slowing down your breath activates your core muscles—which, in turn, allows you to hold this asana. Remain conscious of each exhalation. Note that activating the right set of muscles at the appropriate intensity makes the position feel comfortable and steady.

ADVICE FOR THE PRACTITIONER

Chaturanga dandasana can be challenging to perform at first, until your arms, back the and legs become strong enough to support you. From the plank pose (refer to its description as part of asana 3 under 'yoga for mother and child'), begin by lowering your knees to the mat and then, with an exhalation, lower your sternum within an inch or two above the mat.

PARTNERING

Your partner can observe you as you assume the pose and provide feedback, which can help you keep your heels, knees, hip girdle and shoulders in one line. Your partner can also encourage you to take long, deep breaths by paying attention to the sound of your respiration. Lastly, your partner can also ease your back and give you a gentle massage when you come out of the pose.

VARIATIONS

Once you're comfortable in chaturanga dandasana, you could attempt the following variation.

Suggested variation: Lift your right leg up when you are in the push-up position (as described under 'getting into the asana'); balance yourself on your arms and the toes of your left foot. Slowly, lower your body, keeping it just above the mat. Listen to the sound of your breath as your nostrils remain close to the mat. Come out of the pose by lowering the right leg down. Glide your body into adho mukha svanasana or parvatasana (asana 12 under 'the preparatory series'). Switch legs and practise this with the other side.

BENEFITS

Chaturanga dandasana and its variation help:

- strengthen the arms and wrists
- tone the abdomen

CONTRAINDICATIONS AND CAUTIONS

This asana should be avoided if you're battling the carpal tunnel syndrome. Pregnant women, too, should skip this pose.

ASANA 18: NATARAJASANA
(DANCING SHIVA POSE)

METHOD

Getting into the Asana

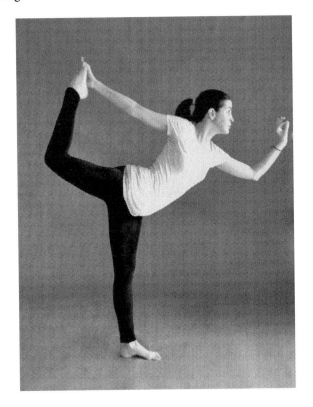

1. Stand tall on the mat with your feet parallel to each other.
2. Shift your body weight to the left foot, bend your right leg and grab the ankle with your right hand.
3. Extend your left arm and make a loop by joining the tip of the index finger with the tip of the thumb (chin mudra).
4. Push your right foot away from the hip and allow your back to arch as you shift your upper body forward.

Maintaining the Asana

1. Hold your left hand and your right foot in line with each other.
2. Keep pushing the heel away from the hip, letting the thigh do all the work; use the entire length of the right arm by keeping it straight and pulled.
3. Breathe in and out, with very soft and slow inhalations and exhalations. Hold the asana for five to eight breaths.

Coming out of the Asana

1. Relax your right thigh and release the ankle, and place the foot back on the mat.
2. Lower your left arm down and come back into the standing position.
3. Repeat the asana with the other side.

MODIFICATIONS

If the hamstrings feel tight, you can gently bend or soften the knee of the balancing leg. This will also help if you have some difficulty maintaining your balance.

OBSERVATIONS

Observe how sending the heel of the raised leg away from the hip activates the right set of muscles and deepens the arch of the back. Also notice how this helps the arm holding it to get pulled, which further opens the chest, allowing each breath to flow deep into the lungs. Note how fixing the gaze at one point and maintaining slow inhalations and exhalations improves your overall sense of balance. Besides, note how letting the body weight shift forward by lowering the chest makes the raised leg go higher up and further deepens the arch of the back.

ADVICE FOR THE PRACTITIONER

As you hold the pose with one hand in the chin mudra, fix your gaze at a point and keep looking at it through the loop you are making with your index finger and the thumb. This will allow you to balance yourself more effectively.

PARTNERING

Your partner can simply stay next to you and provide you with any assistance or support you may need to gain or regain the balance whilst getting into or maintaining the asana. Your partner can also encourage you with carefully chosen words of praise.

VARIATIONS

Once you're comfortable in natarajasana, you could attempt the following variation.

Suggested variation: After getting into the asana (as described above), continue to hold the right foot with the right hand. Send the left arm back and grab the right foot with both the hands. Roll your shoulder blades towards the spine, letting the chest open. Lean your chest forward and lift your chin up.

BENEFITS

Natarajasana and its variation help:

- stretch the shoulders and chest
- stretch the thighs, groin and abdomen

- strengthen the legs and ankles
- improve balance

CONTRAINDICATIONS AND CAUTIONS

This asana should be avoided if you're battling the carpal tunnel syndrome and/or herniated discs. Pregnant women, too, should avoid this pose.

ASANA 19: PADMASANA
(LOTUS POSE)

METHOD

Getting into the Asana

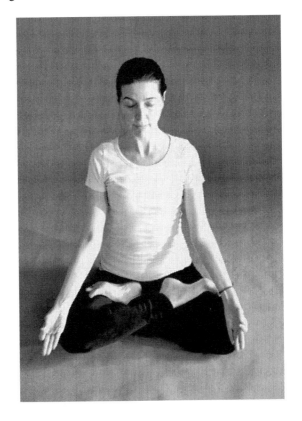

1. Start by sitting on the mat with your legs stretched out in front of you. Bend your right knee and hold the right foot with your right hand, and pull it in towards your abdomen; place it on top of your left leg.
2. Press your right knee towards the mat and grab your left foot; bend the knee and place it on top of the right thigh, very close to the abdomen.
3. Now place both your hands on the knees and press the knees down to the mat.

Maintaining the Asana

1. Keep pushing the knees towards the mat.
2. Keep the arms straight and push them forward to activate your lower back muscles.
3. Pull your chest up and hold an erect back. Maintain the position by keeping the crown of the head pointed upwards.
4. After a few breaths, unlock your feet and switch legs.

Coming out of the Asana

1. Relax your back, use your hands to unlock your feet from their position and stretch out the legs.
2. Shake your legs if you feel any numbness.

MODIFICATIONS

You can bring your first leg in position, as described above, and then, simply slide the lower leg under the upper leg. This is called ardha padmasana (half lotus pose).

OBSERVATIONS

Once you are comfortably settled in the asana, simply observe how the oneness of your legs helps evenly distribute the weight of the body. Notice how, when the legs form a stable base, it becomes relatively easier to hold the spine upright; this has an impact on the flow of breath, which becomes effortless, and the duration of each inhalation and exhalation increases.

ADVICE FOR THE PRACTITIONER

This is one of the most important asanas in yoga because it provides a great stable posture for one to meditate in. Getting padmasana right takes a lot of time, and the aim is to get to a point where the asana can be maintained effortlessly. Some people get into the lotus position in less than a second. Others, though, could struggle, particularly if the hips and the lower back are not very flexible, and the motion of a knee joint comes with hindrances; under such circumstances, the student has to be patient and work with hip openers to build the kind of mobility needed to get into the asana effortlessly. Eventually, s/he will be able to meditate and practise pranayama while seated in padmasana.

PARTNERING

Your partner can help you maintain the upright position of your spine by making sure that you align your chest with your hips.

BENEFITS

Padmasana helps:

- stretch the ankles and knees
- stimulate the pelvis, spine, abdomen and bladder
- ease childbirth, if consistently practised until late into pregnancy
- ease menstrual discomfort and sciatica
- destroy all disease and awaken the kundalini (according to traditional texts)
- calm the brain

CONTRAINDICATIONS AND CAUTIONS

This asana should be avoided if you're battling an ankle and/or a knee injury. Padmasana is viewed as an intermediate/advanced pose. Do not attempt it without sufficient prior experience, and without the supervision of an experienced teacher.

ASANA 20: HALASANA
(PLOUGH POSE)

METHOD

Getting into the Asana

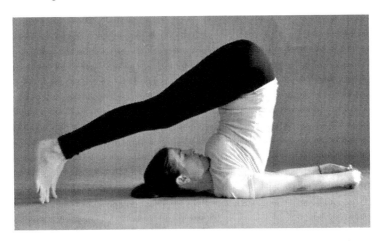

1. Lie down on the mat. Bend your legs, lift your feet and swing your legs up; push them towards the ceiling, pointing the toes up. Support the lower back with both your hands. This is known as sarvangasana or a shoulder-stand.

2. Release your breath and bend your body from the hip joints to slowly lower your toes to the mat. Your legs will be stretched over the head; the toes will be touching the mat; your tailbone will be pointed up; and your weight will rest towards your shoulders. With your toes on the mat and pointed in, keep

the neck in line with the spine; continue to push your chin away from your chest and keep the back of the neck relaxed.

3. Now, very gently, still keeping your body weight towards the shoulders, take the support of your feet, maintain your balance and release your hands away from your back. Stretch your arms out behind you on the mat, in the opposite direction from where your heels are pointing. Interlock your fingers, stretch your arms out and push them into the mat.

4. Squeeze your shoulder blades and press against the mat with your hands to ensure that the tailbone still points towards the ceiling.

Maintaining the Asana

1. Ensure that your body weight remains around your shoulders.
2. Let your fingers remain interlocked and keep the triceps active.
3. Keep the back of your neck long and your chin close to your chest.
4. Hold the pose for ten seconds if you're new to it; increase the duration to a maximum of three minutes once your body is accustomed to the asana.

Coming out of the Asana

1. Release your hands and place them on your lower back with your elbows against the mat.
2. Bend your legs and drop your knees to your ears, keeping the knees slightly away from each other. Look up towards the ceiling.
3. Shift your body weight to your elbows. Lift your knees up and move your thighs so that they are parallel to the floor.
4. Lower your heels closer to your hips and very gently, using the core muscles as brakes, bring the lower back on the mat, vertebra by vertebra.

5. Place your lower back gently on the mat and keep your legs bent.
6. Hold this position for a few breaths as you press your lower back into the mat.

MODIFICATIONS

If your lower back is not very flexible, or you are unable to place your shoulder on the mat when your fingers are interlocked, keep your knees slightly bent.

To begin with, you can practise the pose close to a wall and let your toes touch the wall's surface. Walk your toes down the wall. You can bend your knees, if required. Doing the asana against the wall gives you a sense of balance.

OBSERVATIONS

When coming into this pose, notice how, when you squeeze your shoulder blades together, you lift yourself with the top of your shoulders. Once situated in this position, also notice how when you broaden the shoulder blades across the back, you reduce the resistance of the upper arms.

While holding halasana, make note of the way the back of the spine is stretched.

As you come out of the pose, observe how the vertebrae seem 'open'. Notice the way the body would like to stay curled in. Study how long it takes the spine to stretch back.

ADVICE FOR THE PRACTITIONER

As your legs move over your head, keep your eyes open and your knees wide so the ceiling remains visible. This will allow you to stay oriented and aware of your position.

It can be a bit tricky to take a deep breath when the torso is curled under the weight of the legs, but make sure that you respire effortlessly.

PARTNERING

Your partner should stand close to where your feet will land while in halasana. Perform the pose, and your partner can hold your feet and gently guide you as you bring them down. This assistance is especially helpful when you're coming to grips with how you are to shift your body weight.

Your partner can also assist you by standing with her/his foot between your interlocked arms, and can gently keep a knee on your lower back to provide support; with such pressure, your tailbone climbs up, thus deepening the asana.

VARIATIONS

Once you're comfortable in halasana, you could attempt the following variation.

Suggested variation: Practise halasana by keeping your hands on your back. Release your breath and bend your body from the hip joints to slowly lower your toes to the mat. Point your toes out in such a way that the top of your feet touch the mat. Keep the knees wide open and lower them next to your ears. Relax your legs and let their weight help you maintain the pose effortlessly.

Slowly move the arms over the head, and close to the toes. Wrap your arms around your thighs as though you are hugging them. Grab your wrists, and keep the head comfortably placed in between your knees.

When you are ready to come out of the pose, support your lower back with your palms and steady your elbows on the mat. Lift your legs up one by one and bend both your knees towards your chest; keep your feet close to your hips. Slowly release the support of the lower back and place the spine on the mat as gradually as you can.

BENEFITS

Halasana and its variation help:

- stretch the shoulders and spine
- stimulate the abdominal organs and the thyroid gland
- relieve the symptoms of menopause
- address backaches, headaches, infertility, insomnia and sinusitis
- reduce stress and fatigue
- calm the brain

CONTRAINDICATIONS AND CAUTIONS

This asana should be avoided if you're battling diarrhoea and/or a neck injury. Pregnant or menstruating women, too, should avoid this pose. If you're a patient of asthma and/or high blood pressure, practise halasana with your legs supported by props.

ASANA 21: ARDHA MATSYENDRASANA (HALF LORD OF THE FISHES POSE)

METHOD

Getting into the Asana

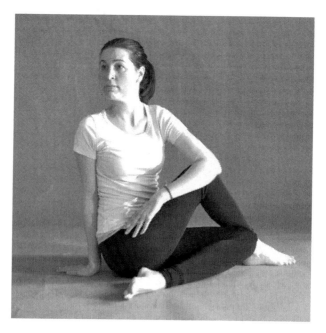

1. Sit on the mat with your legs stretched out in front of you and parallel to each other. Bend your right leg and place your right leg over your left one (which is straight). The right knee will point towards the ceiling.

2. Bring your right arm to your shoulder level and push it back. Lower your right hand and place it very close to your tailbone; push this hand into the mat to get the arm totally straight.

3. Grab your right knee with your left hand and pull it closer to your left shoulder.

4. Now, holding your right knee—which is pointing up and is close to your left shoulder—move your left elbow over your right knee, bringing the right knee under the left arm.

5. Bend your left leg and place your left foot right under your right hip. You could grab your right foot or ankle with your left hand.

Maintaining the Asana

1. Hold your right arm straight and parallel to your spine.

2. Keep your right shoulder away from your ear by lifting your head up.

3. Slow your breath and let each inhalation make its way to the bottom of your lungs.

4. Keep your left elbow pushed into your right knee and hold your right foot with your left arm straight.

5. Keep looking over your right shoulder and watch the way every inhalation lifts your chest and every exhalation rolls the right shoulder further out.

6. Hold the position for ten long, deep breaths.

Coming out of the Asana

1. Release the asana with an exhalation.

2. Stretch your left leg forward.

3. Release the pressure on your right knee and lift your left elbow up to come out of the twist.

4. Stretch your right leg forward and repeat the process with the other side.

MODIFICATIONS

While in the asana (as described above) push your left elbow into your right knee and gain the entire length of the spine to create more space for the spine to twist. Keeping the left arm straight and grabbing the ankle or toes on the right foot locks the asana and makes the grip even tighter.

You can settle your right hip into the arch of your left foot. Rolling the right shoulder blade, twist your upper body and with the right side of the upper back, squeeze the tension out of the muscles.

Also, play around with your right foot. You can slide it away from the hip and give yourself a broader base to settle on. Move your body weight sideways and notice the precise movement that deepens the stretch.

Hold the pose for five to eight breaths. Now, switch the position of the legs.

OBSERVATIONS

Notice how (as part of the sequence under 'getting into the asana') holding the left arm parallel to the spine makes the asana grow even 'taller' since the entire length of the spine is utilized. Sense how rolling of the shoulders massages the muscles between the spine and the shoulder blades.

Also observe the way your breath functions in this asana. Watch the way the chest lifts with every inhalation—making the body want to unwind and come out of the asana. Watch how, when you breathe out, the lungs seem to become flaccid, creating more space inside the torso, and making the body sink further into the twist.

ADVICE FOR THE PRACTITIONER

Pressing the palm of the arm that is behind into the mat will help you keep the spine straight. It will also allow you to roll the shoulder blades better, which in turn, will help you expand the chest further.

PARTNERING

A partner can help you sink deeper into the twist. While following the sequence under 'getting into the asana', have your partner sit near your right side. S/he will hold your right wrist with both hands and can lean back, pulling your arm. Now your partner will lift her/his left leg up, and resting on the buttocks, place her/his foot on your right shoulder. That gives your partner control over the twist. Communicate with your partner and convey the kind of pull or push that is comfortable and appreciated.

Your partner can also help you sink deeper into the twist by sitting right behind you, placing her/his hands on your shoulders and applying gentle pressure in the direction of the twist. You can mimic the sound of your partner's long, deep and slow breath.

VARIATIONS

Once you're comfortable in ardha matsyendrasana, you could attempt the following variation.

Suggested variation: After following the sequence under 'getting into the asana', raise your left arm up and point it up towards the ceiling. Now lower the left hand and dip it between your legs, keeping the hand as close to the torso as possible, with the palm facing outwards.

Now, wrap the right arm around the torso. With the left hand grab the fingers or wrist of the right hand, whichever is comfortable at that point of time. Roll your right shoulder further back to squeeze your shoulders towards your spine. Keep the spine tall and twisted. Make sure that you're breathing consistently.

BENEFITS

Ardha matsyendrasana and its variation help:

- stretch the shoulders, hips and neck
- energize the spine
- stimulate the liver, kidneys and the 'digestive fire' in the belly
- relieve menstrual discomfort, fatigue, sciatica and backaches
- address asthma and infertility
- increase the appetite, destroy most deadly diseases and awaken the kundalini (according to traditional texts)

CONTRAINDICATIONS AND CAUTIONS

This asana should be avoided in case of a back injury and/or any kind of spine aggravation. Attempt this pose only under the supervision of an experienced teacher.

ASANA 22: JANU SIRSASANA (HEAD-TO-KNEE FORWARD BEND)

METHOD

Getting into the Asana

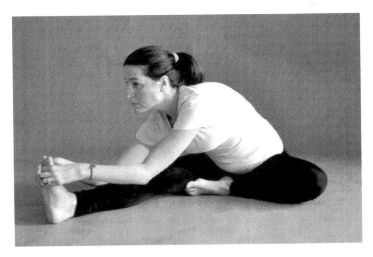

1. Sit on the mat with your legs stretched out in front of you. Use a blanket under your buttocks, if necessary. Take in a long, deep breath, bend your left knee and place the left heel close to your perineum.
2. Rest the sole of your left foot lightly on the inner side of your right thigh, and lower your left knee to the mat, with the shin at a right angle to the right leg. Point the toes of your right foot towards yourself and keep your right heel

pushed out to ensure that the hamstrings of your right leg remain stretched.

3. Reach out with your right hand and grab your right foot, shin or ankle. Release your breath gently and twist your torso slightly to the right, your chest turned towards the mat.

4. Now reach out with your left arm and place your hand on your right wrist. While releasing your breath very gently, curl your head in and lower your chin down towards your chest. Line up your navel with the middle of the right thigh.

5. Hold the asana, keeping the muscles around your neck and shoulders relaxed.

Maintaining the Asana

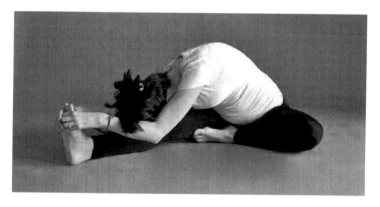

1. Keep breathing in and out, listening to the sound of your breath.

2. Keep your elbows away from each other, so there's space for your head to draw near your knee. Use the weight of your head and the force of gravity to effortlessly keep your body in close proximity to the mat.

3. Keep your eyes closed and maintain the asana for eight to ten long, deep breaths.

Coming out of the Asana

1. Take in a long, deep breath and lift your chest up.
2. Raise your arms so they're in line with your spine and in touch with your ears; hold your spine perpendicular to the floor and keep your shoulders relaxed.
3. Lower your arms.
4. Switch the position of your legs and repeat the asana.

MODIFICATIONS

If you cannot comfortably reach the foot of the extended leg, simply grab your ankle, shin or just the knee. Bending the leg can also be helpful if the stretch feels far too severe.

OBSERVATIONS

Notice that the way you place the foot of your extended leg changes the intensity of the stretch in the hamstrings. If you hold your toes as they point inwards, you are likely to feel a stretch at the back of your knee and your thigh, all the way to your spine. Holding the outer edge of your foot with your hands and keeping your arms totally straight will likely grant you a 'stretch' along the outer side of the extended leg.

ADVICE FOR THE PRACTITIONER

Allow the force of gravity, and the intake and expulsion of air, take the body lower down, towards the mat. Remember that muscles stretch better when they are totally relaxed; if your muscles are tense, it's hard to stretch them.

When your chest and abdomen face down, you get to stretch the sides of the torso more intensely.

PARTNERING

The partner can support you by applying gentle pressure to your lower back; this will help you to fold further, from the base of the spine. S/he can remind you to keep the muscles around your shoulders relaxed.

VARIATIONS

The intensity of the stretch varies, depending on the angle the shin of your bent leg makes with your outstretched leg. Once you're comfortable in janu sirsasana, you could attempt the following variation.

Suggested variation: You can slide the bent knee away from the outstretched leg and reach out with your left hand to grab your right foot (while following the sequence under 'getting into the asana').

BENEFITS

Janu sirsasana and its variation help:

- stretch the spine, shoulders, hamstrings and groin
- stimulate the liver and kidneys
- strengthen the back muscles during pregnancy, up to the second trimester (in such a situation, the asana should be attempted without coming forward, while keeping the spine concave and front torso long)
- improve digestion
- address high blood pressure, insomnia and sinusitis
- relieve the symptoms of menopause
- relieve anxiety, fatigue, headaches and menstrual discomfort
- calm the brain and relieve mild depression

CONTRAINDICATIONS AND CAUTIONS

This asana should be avoided if you're battling asthma; diarrhoea; and/or a knee injury.

ASANA 23: SUPTA BADDHA KONASANA (RECLINING BOUND ANGLE POSE)

METHOD

Getting into the Asana

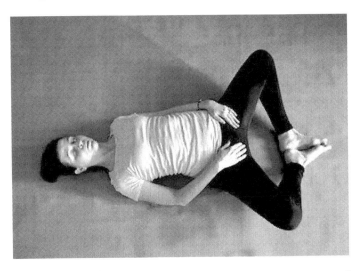

1. Get into savasana (asana 11 under 'the preparatory series'). Bend your legs and put the soles of your feet together.
2. Drop your knees down and away from each other towards the mat. Allow your legs and your entire body to relax.
3. Reduce the arch in your lower back by pressing the lumbar area into the mat, and by curling in the tailbone.

4. Keep your elbows next to your body and place your hands on top of your abdomen. Focus on your breath.

Maintaining the Asana

1. Keep your head in line with your spine, with your chin lowered towards your chest.
2. Keep your inner thighs relaxed and let your knees feel heavy. Keep your arms relaxed, too, and lay them down by the sides of your body. All the muscles are now at ease, with no engagement of muscular strength.
3. Keep your breaths slow and long for about a minute.

Coming out of the Asana

1. Use your hands to press your thighs together, then roll over to one side.
2. Push yourself away from the mat, your head trailing your torso.

MODIFICATIONS

If your inner thighs feel far too stretched and relaxing the muscles of the thighs becomes even more painful, place two cushions under both your thighs to support them. This will allow you to enjoy the 'stretch', while remaining comfortable in the asana.

OBSERVATIONS

Notice how the weight of the knees allows you to sink deeper into the asana. Also notice how relaxing the inside of your thighs makes your knees feel heavy.

Avoid struggling with the asana by using your strength. Simply let go of the stiffness that pervades your thighs and watch your knees lower down with their own weight, impelled by the force of gravity.

Notice how your breath slows down, and the warm body

opens up. Watch as the navel goes up and down while you lie back and breathe effortlessly.

ADVICE FOR THE PRACTITIONER

You can hold this pose for a long time. Use this opportunity to slip into a round of meditation. Simply lean back, place your palms on your navel and enjoy the rhythm and the pace of your breath.

PARTNERING

Let your partner sit on her/his knees by your head and interlock her/his fingers behind your neck. S/he can lift your head up off the mat by a few centimetres and very gently make your head turn from one side to the next. This will help you relax the back of the neck and the muscles between your shoulder blades.

BENEFITS

Supta baddha konasana helps:

- stretch the inner thighs, groin and knees
- stimulate the abdominal organs like the ovaries and prostate gland, bladder and kidneys
- stimulate the heart and improve general circulation
- address the symptoms of menstruation or menopause
- relieve the symptoms of stress and mild depression

CONTRAINDICATIONS AND CAUTIONS

This asana should be avoided if you're battling a groin injury; a knee injury; and/or lower back issues.

ASANA 24: VRIKSHASANA (TREE POSE)

METHOD

Getting into the Asana

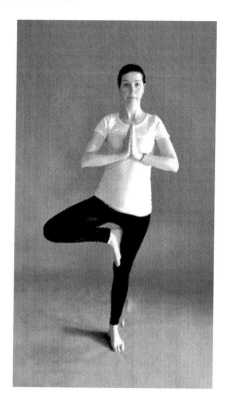

1. Stand with your feet parallel to one another and hip-width apart; divide your body weight equally.
2. Look at a point that is slightly higher than your eye level.
3. Slowly shift your body weight to the left and place your right foot up on the left thigh, with the right heel placed close to the perineum.
4. Join your palms together towards the middle of the chest.
5. Take long, deep and effortless breaths.

Maintaining the Asana

1. Keep pressing your palms into each other.
2. Keep your shoulders relaxed. Your gaze should remain fixed at the point that is slightly higher than the level of your eyes.
3. Maintain the posture with the torso lifted and the toes spread out; this will help lengthen the spine and stabilize the position.
4. Maintain a slow flow of the breath; try holding the pose for about eight rounds of inhaling and exhaling.

Coming out of the Asana

1. Keeping your gaze fixed to maintain your balance, slowly lift your right foot off your left thigh and place it on the mat.
2. Lower your arms down and relax.
3. Repeat the same set of instructions for the other side.

MODIFICATIONS

While following the instructions listed under 'getting into the asana', your right foot can be placed close to your left knee or your left shin or even at the level of the left ankle, with the toes touching the mat. You can bring your arms up over your head and join your hands together. Close your eyes to make this asana more challenging and fun, while visualizing the contact point between your foot and the mat and trying to maintain your balance for as long as possible.

OBSERVATIONS

This pose speaks volumes not only about the state of your physical balance, but also about your emotional and mental equilibrium. Standing quietly on one foot is not as easy as it sounds. Notice how fixing your gaze on the wall in front of you makes maintaining your balance far easier—this is because your brain gets constant feedback from the immediate surroundings and feels oriented.

ADVICE FOR THE PRACTITIONER

The body takes some time to get used to balancing poses. If balancing poses a problem, avoid making the body 'tight' and don't stiffen the muscles. Rather, allow them to relax. To further ease yourself into the pose, distract yourself by focusing on the flow or the sound of breath, instead of trying to balance on one foot. This, in itself, will grant your body greater stability. Now, try remaining calm and holding the pose with acceptance.

Vrikshasana is the foundation of all the balancing asanas. You grow increasingly confident as you practise it regularly.

PARTNERING

Your partner can help you gain and maintain balance if you find vrikshasana challenging. S/he can stand behind you and gently place her/his index finger on the upper part of your spine, right between the shoulder blades, without applying too much pressure. The contact point with your partner will become a point of reference for your brain, making it easier for you to maintain your balance.

VARIATIONS

Once you're comfortable in vrikshasana, you could attempt the following variations.

Variation 1: Vrikshasana can be practised by placing the bent foot further up, close to the hip girdle. This makes the knee of the leg that is lifted up point down towards the mat. You can also wrap the arm corresponding to the lifted-up leg around the waist and grip the toes of the raised foot.

Variation 2: Another variation involves lying down on your back. If seen from above, the asana will appear nearly identical to the pose we've highlighted in the image; however, this variation removes the challenge of maintaining balance.

BENEFITS

Vrikshasana and its first variation help:

- strengthen the muscles surrounding the spine and the buttocks
- improve balance
- improve coordination and brain functioning
- enhance the sense of proprioception
- increase concentration and focus
- improve blood circulation
- strengthen the foundation for advanced balancing yogic asanas

CONTRAINDICATIONS AND CAUTIONS

This asana should be avoided if you're battling knee injuries and/ or vertigo.

ASANA 25: RAJAKAPOTASANA (ONE-LEGGED PIGEON POSE)

METHOD`

Getting into the Asana

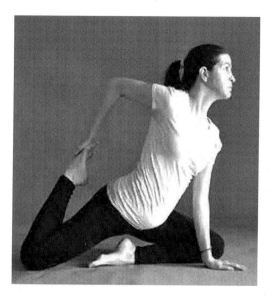

1. Get into adho mukha svanasana or parvatasana (asana 12 under 'the preparatory series').
2. Bend your left leg and bring that knee under your chest.
3. Place the knee down on the mat, keeping the right leg stretched out behind and close to the mat.
4. Lower the hips towards the mat.

5. Firmly press your left palm into the mat and bend the right leg behind. Hold your right ankle with your right hand. Pull your right foot in closer to the hip.

Maintaining the Asana

1. Keep your right heel pushed away from your hip to deepen the arch in your lower back.
2. Keep your hips firm and your chest open.
3. Firmly push your left palm into the mat to maintain the height of the asana or come on the fingertips of the left hand to deepen the arch of the lower back.
4. Focus on each intake of breath, allowing it to expand your chest. Hold on for three to six breaths.

Coming out of the Asana

1. Gently release the ankle you hold and let the right leg stretch down towards the mat.
2. Bring your right hand down to where the left one is. Press both your palms firmly into the mat, lift the hips up and step back with your left leg, your toes keeping pace. Continue to lift your hips towards the ceiling. Bring your body into adho mukha svanasana or parvatasana (asana 12 under 'the preparatory series').
3. Lower your knees slowly and fold the body into shashankasana (asana 9 under 'the preparatory series').
4. Stay here for a few breaths to relax the spine completely; then come up gently.
5. Repeat the same set of instructions for the other side.

MODIFICATIONS

If you are flexible, you can slide the foot of the bent leg (the leg in front) behind the opposite hand. This will increase the stretch along your hip.

OBSERVATIONS

Observe how—while following the sequence under 'getting into the asana'—as you come on your left fingertips and pull your chest away from your left knee, your spine lengthens. Feel the muscles surrounding your spine, especially those around your lower back, getting activated and notice how they hold the torso firm. Observe your hips as they sink down and your chest as it goes up. Note whether you feel any stretch along the back of your thigh when the leg is bent.

ADVICE FOR THE PRACTITIONER

There are several graceful variations for this position, but for some individuals it might take a period of long and regular practice to achieve the most advanced of poses associated with rajakapotasana. Do not get discouraged. What's important is for the asana is to 'feel' graceful, no matter what the level of flexibility is.

PARTNERING

The partner can stay behind you and firmly place her/his hands on your shoulders, so that you can lift your hands off the mat. From this position, you can wrap your hands around your partner's neck, thus lengthening your spine considerably. The support of your partner will also give you the opportunity to deepen the arch in your lower back.

VARIATIONS

Once you're comfortable in rajakapotasana, you could attempt the following variations.

Variation 1: While following the sequence under 'getting into the asana', bend the outstretched leg behind, pointing the foot towards the ceiling. Balancing on your left palm, stretch your right arm out and grab your right foot. Pull this foot closer to the hip to deepen the stretch in the right thigh.

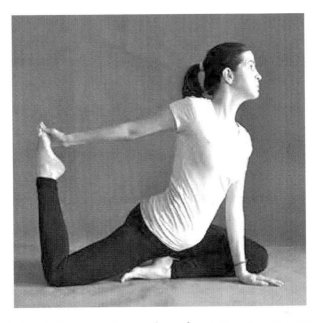

Variation 2: Once you have achieved variation 1, you can wrap your right arm around the right foot in such a way that the top of the foot rests between your forearm and the biceps while the heel touches your right buttock.

Variation 3: From variation 2, stretch the right arm behind, letting the foot slip into the hand. Use the strength of your right thigh to send your heel away from your hip. You will notice that your right arm gets pulled. Moreover, the arch in your back will also deepen.

Variation 4: Taking off variation 3, place your right big toe loosely between your thumb and the index and middle fingers of your right hand. As you pull this foot closer to your hip, rotate your right elbow clockwise in such a way that your elbow ends up pointing towards the ceiling, even while the foot remains in your hand. Keeping your lower back muscles active (while ensuring that the torso is upright and balanced), lift your left arm off the mat and grab the right big toe with both your hands. If your flexibility levels permit this, drop your head back and let the crown of your head touch the sole of your right foot.

BENEFITS

Rajakapotasana and its variations help:

- strengthen the arms
- strengthen the back and the thigh
- open the hips and the chest
- increase the flexibility of the lower body
- expand the lungs, promoting deep inhalation

CONTRAINDICATIONS AND CAUTIONS

This pose is to be avoided if you're battling a herniated or slipped disc, and/or injuries, since it puts pressure on the knees and the ankles.

ASANA 26: VIRABHADRASANA (WARRIOR POSE)

METHOD

Getting into the Asana

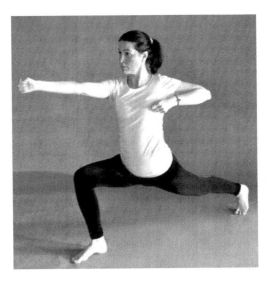

1. Stand straight with the arms along the body. Release your breath, take your left foot back and place the toes on the mat; keep the left knee off the mat and pointing towards the floor. Stretch your arms out forward, parallel to each other and to the floor.

2. Turn your left foot slightly to the left. Keep your right foot to the right at a 90-degree angle; your right thigh will be parallel to the floor. Keep your left heel off the mat and pushed outwards,

away from your body, to distribute your body weight evenly in order to avoid straining the right thigh in front.

3. Release your breath and bend your right knee such that it is over your right ankle—so that the shin is perpendicular to the floor. Lower your hips to get your right thigh parallel to the floor. Anchor the movement of the right knee by strengthening your left leg and pressing the outer left heel firmly into the mat.

4. Pull your left arm back as if you are pulling an arrow. Hold your elbow at shoulder level. Maintain a gentle lift in the chest. Keep the sides of your torso equally long and your shoulders directly over your pelvis. Press your tailbone slightly towards the pubis. Look towards the spot that your right hand is pointing at.

Maintaining the Asana

1. Keep breathing in and out, slowly and effortlessly.
2. Hold this position for five to seven long, deep breaths.

Coming out of the Asana

1. Inhale to come up.
2. Reverse your feet and repeat for the same number of breaths, switching the position of your legs.

MODIFICATIONS

If you have difficulty supporting yourself in this pose (as described under 'getting into the asana'), practise virabhadrasana with a wall behind you and press your left heel against the wall. This will help you anchor the pose.

OBSERVATIONS

To increase the length and strength of the arms in the pose, turn the palms and inner elbow creases, such that they face the ceiling, while you draw your shoulder blades towards the back.

Then, while maintaining the rotation of your arms, turn your palms from around the wrist-area to face the floor again.

ADVICE FOR THE PRACTITIONER

When you bend your right knee at a right angle while following the instructions under 'getting into the asana', ensure that you bend it very quickly with a loud exhalation, and aim the inside of the right knee at the little-toe side of the right foot.

PARTNERING

A partner can help you stabilize the asana by standing behind you and helping you anchor the leg at the back.

Alternatively, your partner could stand right behind you as your back leg passes between her/his legs. Send both your arms up and back till your hands are behind your partner's neck, and interlock your fingers. Now, as your partner stands tall, you can relax your front leg and allow your hips to sink low; you'll feel your arms lengthening and receive amazing support along the way!

VARIATIONS

Once you feel comfortable in virabhadrasana, you could attempt the following variation.

Suggested variation: Maintaining the asana, as described under 'getting into the asana', point your right arm up as if you are aiming the bow and arrow towards the sky. Pull your chest back, away from the knee in front, letting your body deepen the arch. Lower your hips down to ensure that the thigh in front remains parallel to the floor. Keep your eyes open and breathe normally. Repeat with the opposite side.

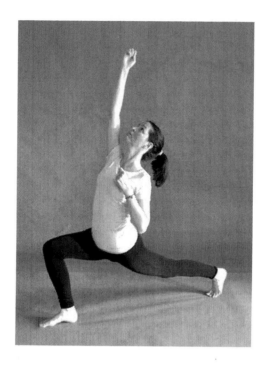

BENEFITS

Virbhadrasana and its variation help:

- strengthen and stretch the legs and ankles
- stretch the groin, chest, lungs and shoulders
- stimulate the abdominal organs
- increase stamina
- relieve backaches, especially through the second trimester of pregnancy
- address the carpal tunnel syndrome, flat feet, infertility, osteoporosis and sciatica

CONTRAINDICATIONS AND CAUTIONS

This asana should be avoided if you're battling diarrhoea and/or high blood pressure.

If you have neck problems, don't turn your head; continue to look straight ahead with both sides of the neck of equal length.

ASANA 27: PURVOTTANASANA (REVERSE PLANK POSE)

METHOD

Getting into the Asana

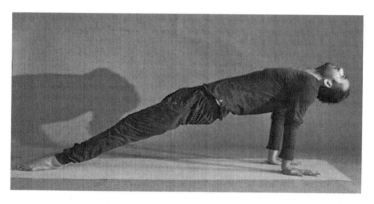

1. Sit on the mat with your legs outstretched in front of you. Place your arms behind on the mat, with the fingers pointing away from the body. The width between the hands will be slightly narrower than that between the shoulder blades.
2. Stretch the feet and point the toes towards the mat. Start pressing into the mat with your palms. Keep looking towards your toes. Use your lower back and the muscles of the buttocks to push your body up, until your toes, ankles, knees, hip girdle and shoulders are in one line.
3. Slowly drop your head back until your throat is in line with your spine. Keep your lips pursed and your eyes open.

4. Focus on your breath and allow each inhalation to become slow and deep.

Maintaining the Asana

1. Squeeze the buttocks to make the asana firm.
2. Squeeze the shoulder blades in towards the spine to expand the chest and allow each breath to sink deeper into the lungs.
3. Keep your head dropped back and your chin pointed out to maintain a stretch along the front of your neck. Hold on for thirty seconds.

Coming out of the Asana

1. Lower your chin and look towards your toes.
2. Relax your lower back and the hips and slowly lower yourself down on the mat.

MODIFICATIONS

You can keep your fingers pointed in rather than outwards. Explore what works better for you.

OBSERVATIONS

Observe how, in this position, your body is so straight that your toes, ankles, knees, hips and shoulders are in a single line; since your chin points out, your throat is in line with the spine.

Also notice that in this asana, your breath becomes effortless and long.

ADVICE FOR THE PRACTITIONER

Keep your eyes open while performing this asana if you find it hard to maintain your balance. Squeezing the buttocks will help you lift your body further up and grant you greater stability.

PARTNERING

Have your partner stand near your feet. Once you are up in purvottanasana, your partner can push your toes down into the mat; this will help align the joints and lift your body further up.

VARIATIONS

Once you're comfortable in purvottanasana, you could attempt the following variations.

Variation 1: While holding purvottanasana and maintaining the height of the hips, lift your right leg up until your toes are at the level of your eyes. Repeat this with the other side.

Variation 2: Holding purvottanasana, keep your feet half a metre apart. From here, turn both your feet towards the right. Slowly, get the weight off of your left hand and raise your left arm up towards the ceiling. Your torso is gently twisted towards the right. To come out of this pose, place your left arm down in the initial position. Point the toes up towards the ceiling and bring the hips down towards the mat. Repeat the sequence with the other side.

BENEFITS

Purvottanasana and its variations help:

- strengthen the arms, the lower back, upper back, the thighs and the buttocks
- stretch the pectorals and open the chest

CONTRAINDICATIONS AND CAUTIONS

This asana should be avoided if you're battling any spine-related issue (slipped or herniated disc) and/or wrist or ankle injuries.

If you suffer from vertigo, avoid dropping your head back.

ASANA 28:
KAKASANA (CROW POSE)

METHOD

Getting into the Asana

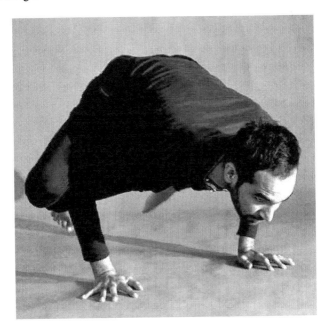

1. Squat down on the mat.
2. Place your hands on the mat, under your shoulders, with your fingers spread open and wide.
3. Point your elbows towards the inside of your knees. Bend

your arms gently, pushing the knees away from each other with the help of your elbows and bringing your body's weight towards your palms.

4. Lift your chin up, while getting the spine straight.
5. Lift your hips up; this will further release the weight off the toes, preparing them, so they lift off the mat.
6. Lift the toes off the mat one by one and maintain your balance, keeping the chin pointed out while looking towards the mat.

Maintaining the Asana

1. Keep inhaling and exhaling slowly without any sort of breath retention.
2. Keep the core muscles active.
3. You may have to adjust the position of your head (shift it upwards or downwards) to ensure that your weight is appropriately distributed; this will allow you to maintain your balance.

Coming out of the Asana

1. Lift the chin up and away from the chest. This will shift your body weight towards the back.
2. Your toes will gently land on the mat.

MODIFICATIONS

Keep your hands wide apart for a broader base for your body to balance. When you are up in the asana, you can let your elbows push your knees away from each other. This will let your body shift closer to the mat—making it easier for you to balance yourself and also, granting greater stability to the posture.

OBSERVATIONS

Observe how the weight of the head plays an important role in this asana. When you lower your chin towards your chest, your body weight shifts forward. When you pull your chin away from your chest by looking up, the body weight goes back towards the feet. As you play around with this, look out for the perfect distribution of weight that will let you maintain your balance effortlessly. The position may look challenging at first, but once you find your centre of balance, it will become easy to stay up there!

ADVICE FOR THE PRACTITIONER

If you are a beginner, you can start practising this asana on a relatively soft surface (a thick mat, for instance), to gain in confidence and build muscle memory.

PARTNERING

Your partner can assist you by making you feel secure. Have your partner stand on the mat, in the direction you are leaning towards. Her/his feet will be as wide as your shoulders are. Once you lean forward, your head can go between your partner's shins and the top of your shoulders can be in touch with your partner's legs. Such support will give you a sense of balance before attempting the asana on your own.

VARIATIONS

Once you feel comfortable in kakasana, you could attempt the following variation.

Suggested variation: You can join your knees and slide both of them towards the outer side of the right elbow, such that your right elbow pushes against the outer side of your left knee. Picture your knees together and your spine twisted. Bend your arms and lean the weight of your upper torso diagonally towards your left hand. Ensure that your feet are still off the mat. Maintain your balance.

BENEFITS

Kakasana and its variation help:

- strengthen the body
- improve a sense of balance
- improve coordination

CONTRAINDICATIONS AND CAUTIONS

This pose should be avoided if you suffer from injured wrists and/or vertigo.

ASANA SEQUENCES IN PARTNER YOGA

After attempting the preparatory series of asanas, you are ready for partner yoga. In this section, the early asanas that form building blocks are systematically listed. You are also taught how to get into a posture with your partner, maintain it and come out of it, so the transition is smooth and does not cause any injury to either person. Besides this, the ideas guiding the poses—the benefits, the couple dynamics and the biomechanics—are elucidated. Finally, by placing an emphasis on the combined rhythm of the practitioners' respiration, or the stretch offered to specific body parts, every asana attempts to build awareness. Remember, end every asana by slipping into savasana (asana 11 under 'the preparatory series').

Now, you are ready to hit the yoga mat. Get your partner along, smile at one another and have fun!

ASANA 1:
OPENING OM

PREPARATORY ASANA
Sukhasana (asana 14)

METHOD

Getting into the Asana

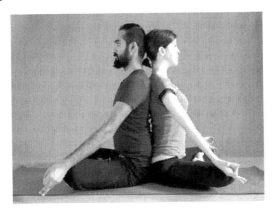

Get ready to start your partner yoga session by chanting the universal sound of 'Om' thrice.

1. Sit on the mat back-to-back with your partner in sukhasana.
2. Keep the spine upright and straight; your spine should be parallel to your partner's, and touching it.
3. Ensure that the head is in a straight line with the spine. The hips and the back of your head should be in touch with those of your partner.

4. Let the hands rest on the knees; your fingers will be in the chin mudra (with the thumb and index finger touching each other).
5. Keep the eyes gently closed.
6. Focus on slowing down your breath, while paying attention to the sound of your partner's inhalation and exhalation, and the gentle pressure exerted on your back by her/his back.
7. Take in a long, deep breath and chant 'Om', keeping the sound protracted and sonorous, and at the same frequency as your partner's voice.
8. Chant 'Om' thrice and relish its powerful sound.
9. At the end of the third 'Om', each partner rubs her/his palms individually, covering the eyes and then slowly opening them.

THE IDEA GUIDING THE ASANA

This opening chant helps set the mood for yoga practice. It makes you aware of your breath and your partner's via the pressure perceived along the spine (as you are sitting back-to-back with someone else).

This asana also gently introduces the element of touch—especially when the partners are not lovers, but friends or colleagues. It is the first opportunity offered to get familiar and comfortable with a yoga partner's touch.

AWARENESS

Become increasingly aware of the sensations along your back, as it remains in touch with your partner's. Notice how the two spines are supporting each other, and that this makes holding the position effortless. Also notice how your back is gently massaged by your partner's breath with every inhalation and exhalation. Tune into the vibrations along the spine, produced by the sound of 'Om', and visualize the chakras running along its length.

ASANA 2:
SEATED SPINAL TWIST

PREPARATORY ASANAS
Bharadvajasana (asana 1)
Ardha matsyendrasana (asana 21)

METHOD

Getting into the Asana

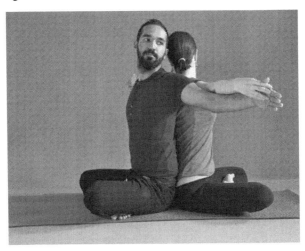

1. Sit back-to-back with your partner on the mat, with your hips, spines and shoulders touching.
2. Raise your arms to your shoulder level. Wrap your arms around those of your partner.
3. While maintaining the back-to-back alignment, both of you

must twist your respective spines towards the right and look over your right shoulders.

4. Press your right shoulder blade against your partner's shoulder, and use the grip and leverage of the intertwined arms to 'deepen the twist' in the spine.

5. Breathe into the twisted spine, while also paying attention to your partner's breath and the resistance of her/his twisted upper body against your back.

6. Change direction and look over your left shoulder by twisting towards the other side, as shown in the image.

Maintaining the Asana

1. Hold the spine straight and keep your arms wrapped around your partner's. Maintain a gentle twist.

2. Breathe in deep. The more you twist, the more your partner is encouraged to follow suit and vice versa. Try holding the pose for thirty seconds.

Coming out of the Asana

1. Release the arms.

2. Stretch the legs out and relax.

THE IDEA GUIDING THE ASANA

The aim is to begin partner yoga with simple poses—those that help you glean the role movement plays in two-person asanas. This one grants a gentle twist to the spine.

AWARENESS

Observe how the movement of the arms can control the twist being offered to the spine, and how the strength applied by one partner can influence the depth of the other partner's twist. Also notice how the muscles of the upper back get squeezed in the twist, and how this helps release the tension around the neck.

ASANA 3:
ADVANCED SPINAL TWIST

PREPARATORY ASANA
Bharadvajasana (asana 1)

METHOD

Getting into the Asana

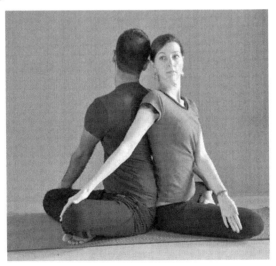

1. Maintain the twist of the previous asana ('seated spinal twist').
2. You can now lower your right hand to the left knee of your partner, and the partner can, similarly, lower her/his right hand to your left knee.

3. Place your left hand on your own right knee; the partner will, likewise, place her/his left hand on her/his right knee.

Maintaining the Asana

1. Use your partner's upper body for leverage, so the weight of your body is counterbalanced. Twist your spine deeply using your arms' strength.
2. Ensure that your breath reaches the bottom of your lungs—enhancing, as a result, the twist and the stretch. As you breathe deep into your twisted body, observe your partner's breath, too.
3. The more you twist, the more your partner will have to twist (and vice versa).
4. Observe your partner's reactions and the comfort level each of you establishes while maintaining a twisted upper body in the asana.
5. Adjust and control the intensity of the twist as well as the leverage of your hands and your partner's, as they push into the knee; ensure that the asana is comfortable for both of you. Both should be able to enjoy the twist and the stretch, while the intake and release of breath remains easy. Try holding the pose for thirty seconds.

Coming out of the Asana

1. Your partner and you will release your arms.
2. Your partner and you can stretch your legs out and relax.

THE IDEA GUIDING THE ASANA

The asana aims to establish both verbal and physical communication between your partner and you while both of you are looking away from each other.

Even as you lead each other to new levels of a twist, the pectorals will open and lengthen along the right side. Moreover, by practising this pose, your spine (and your partner's) will become supple, which will certainly help complete the upcoming asanas in the series.

AWARENESS

Observe how the two of you are linked—each partner has control over the spinal twist of the other; each experiences the impact of the effort the other puts into the twist.

Also observe how by modulating the strength you apply, the depth of the twist varies.

Continue focusing on your connection with your partner as you respire. Since you're back-to-back with your partner, you'll not only experience your breath flowing along your spine, but also your partner's breath flowing along her/his spine.

ASANA 4:
BEYOND THE BUTTERFLY POSE

PREPARATORY ASANAS
Baddha konasana (asana 4)
Sukhasana (asana 14)
Ardha matsyendrasana (asana 21)

METHOD

Getting into the Asana

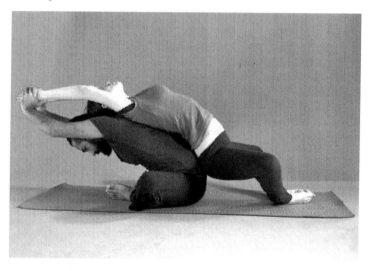

1. Sit back-to-back with your partner and keep the spine
    upright.

2. Ease your respective bodies into baddha konasana.
3. Raise your arms and join hands with your partner.
4. Hold the wrist of your partner and bend forward.
5. Your partner gently lifts her/his hips off the mat and, keeping her/his spine in close contact with yours, s/he leans on your back—the intensity of the back arches of both the partners will match.

Maintaining the Asana

1. After following the sequence under 'getting into the asana', pull the arms of your partner, so that s/he can feel a stretch in the arms, the back and the inner thighs.
2. Allow yourself to deepen the forward bend with every exhalation, using the weight of the partner. Try holding the pose for thirty seconds.

Coming out of the Asana

1. After following the sequence under 'getting into the asana' and 'maintaining the asana', communicate with your partner to come out of the asana.
2. When you are ready, pull your torso back and let the buttocks of your partner touch the mat.
3. Release the wrists of the partner and both of you can lower your arms.
4. Now, repeat this asana, flipping roles.

THE IDEA GUIDING THE ASANA

This asana promotes deep inhalation and expands the walls of the lungs. It also inculcates a spirit of co-existence.

If you're the one below: You get to enjoy an assisted forward bend.

If you're the one above: You are allowed to let go and experience a backward bend. This posture will lengthen your spine while your arms are pulled and your hips are lifted off the mat. It also helps open the shoulders.

AWARENESS

Notice how comfortable this asana is for your partner and you; this is because both backs arch evenly.

If you're the one below: Observe how having your partner on your back does not feel as heavy as you would have anticipated. Besides, you'll experience, at once, a sense of pride and responsibility as your partner leans on you.

If you're the one above: Notice how comforting it is to be assisted with a backward bend.

ASANA 5:
CHURNING THE MILL POSE

PREPARATORY ASANA
Janu sirsasana (asana 22)

METHOD

Getting into the Asana

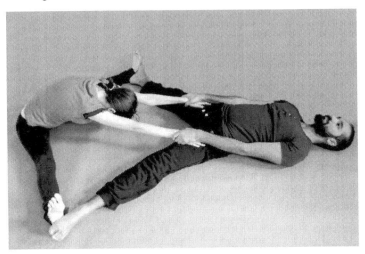

1. Sit down, facing your partner. Stretch your legs out wide in conjunction with her/him.
2. Put your feet against your partner's, hold each other's wrists and look into each other's eyes.

3. Lean back, pulling your partner forward, making sure that both your partner and you have your arms parallel to the floor.
4. Both your partner and you will keep your arms and legs as straight as possible.
5. Make sure that you verbally communicate with your partner. Lean back only as much as your partner finds comfortable. Your partner receives a forward bend.

Maintaining the Asana

1. Alternate bending forward and leaning back, so that both of you rotate clockwise, 'churning the mill' together. Repeat this eight times.
2. Switch roles, with the second partner taking control and leading the 'churning of the mill'. This time ensure that the rotation is anti-clockwise.

Coming out of the Asana

To come out of the asana, return to the centre of the mat and gently release the hands of your partner. Note: Make sure that your partner is stable before letting her/his hands go.

THE IDEA GUIDING THE ASANA

This is a fun exercise. Both of you take turns to stretch each another and challenge one another's flexibility.

In this asana, both of you will look at each other and will, therefore, be able to anticipate any sign of discomfort in the other—which can be addressed by adjusting the intensity of the pull.

This asana helps both of you stretch the hamstrings; work on the potential of the forward bend; open the hips; support the pelvic area; activate the abdominal muscles; warm up the muscles and stretch them; and enhance coordination.

AWARENESS

Observe the reaction of your body and your mind as your partner and you alternate taking control, moving together, and creating and re-creating the motions of churning.

Experience how a physically challenging asana becomes relatively easier when performed in conjunction with a partner; this is because when you're practising as a joint entity, you share the effort in pulling, leaning and churning, which, in turn, grants the pose stability.

Finally, the asana demands that you pay attention to your coordination with your partner.

ASANA 6:
RIDING THE BOAT POSE

PREPARATORY ASANA
Naukasana (asana 3)

METHOD

Getting into the Asana

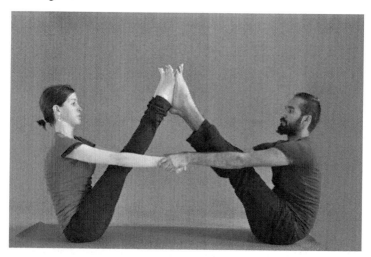

1. Get into naukasana along with your partner.
2. Now, face your partner while maintaining the pose. Your legs can bend slightly and your toes will press against your partner's toes.

3. Reach out with your arms and hold your partner's hands.
4. Lift your right leg up while your partner lifts her/his left leg up. Repeat this with the other leg, too.
5. Balance and stretch the legs till both pairs are straight and the heels are joined.
6. Both of you should push your chests forward, increasing the stretch in the hamstrings.

Maintaining the Asana

1. Keep the legs straight.
2. Keep holding your partner's hand and pulling her/him gently, while keeping the chest lifted.
3. Hold the spine upright.
4. Keep breathing. Try holding the pose for thirty seconds.

Coming out of the Asana

1. Coming out of this asana is fun, too. Maintain the grip of your partner's wrists and soften the knees. This will allow you to unlock the position.
2. From here, both of you will lower the feet down at the same pace and your heels will touch the mat at the same time.
3. Release the wrists of your partner and relax.

THE IDEA GUIDING THE ASANA

This asana helps stretch the legs and activate the muscles surrounding the spine.

It also improves your ability to maintain balance by using your core strength and by responding to the movements of your partner.

AWARENESS

Notice the involvement of the core of the body to maintain this posture. Experience the way two bodies counterbalance each other. Focus on a soothing sensation, as the soles of your partner's feet touch your soles. When they press against each other, they help you keep your back straight and maintain your balance; the partner will feel the same way.

ASANA 7:
BIGGER BOAT POSE

PREPARATORY ASANAS
Naukasana (asana 3)
Virabhadrasana (asana 26)

METHOD

Getting into the Asana

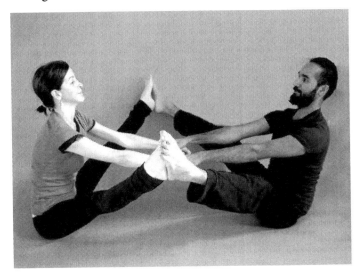

1. Get into the previous asana ('riding the boat pose').
2. Bend your legs, and lower your feet down in line with your shoulders, making sure you are keeping your soles pressed

with your partner's.

3. While you maintain your balance, continue holding your partner's hands, as both of you bring your arms together inside the legs.
4. Use core strength so that both of you can straighten your legs together and let your legs go wide at the same time.
5. Push the chest forward and upwards.

Maintaining the Asana

1. Firmly keep the soles of your feet pressed with the partner's.
2. Ensure that your legs remain straight.
3. Use the strength of your legs to keep them stable in the prescribed position.
4. Look into each other's eyes and pretend that it's an easy pose, while attempting to hold it for thirty seconds.

Coming out of the Asana

1. In order to come out of the asana, gently coordinate the next steps with your partner. Bend your knees and lower your feet down on the mat very gently.
2. Release the hands.

THE IDEA GUIDING THE ASANA

Though this asana looks similar to the previous one, it revolves around a completely different set of dynamics. It actively engages the thigh and core muscles.

To maintain your balance and breathe properly, while holding this physically challenging posture, you will need to coordinate your movements with your partner. Both of you need to adapt; each needs to adjust to the other's ability to stretch and balance/counterbalance, pushing and pulling all along to keep the back straight and the legs up.

AWARENESS

Notice the equilibrium and the balance that two bodies achieve by working together. Compare this with the counterbalance offered by the previous asana.

Experience the support given by the push-and-pull between your partner and you.

Become aware of the gentle flow of your breath as you engage your muscles—keeping your legs up and unbent, your core active and your back straight.

ASANA 8:
PARALLEL PLANKS POSE

PREPARATORY ASANAS
Chaturanga dandasana (asana 17)
Purvottanasana (asana 27)

METHOD

Getting into the Asana

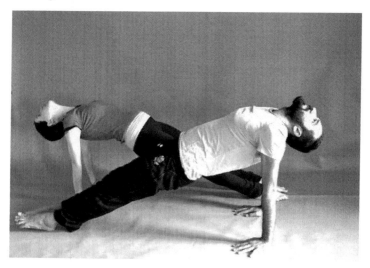

1. Sit on the mat with your legs straight and extended forward.
    Keep your back straight.
2. Keep your arms placed along your body, your hands in line

with your hips, and the fingers pointing out.

3. Lift your hips off the mat (as much as is possible), keeping your legs straight and your feet spread on the mat.

4. Lift your chin up and look back.

5. Your partner follows the same set of instructions and, facing you, gets into the same pose.

6. To come out of the posture, bring your chin towards the chest first, then bring the hips back to the mat and relax.

Maintaining the Asana

1. Visualize your toes, ankles, knees, hip joints and shoulders in one line with each other.

2. Squeeze the buttocks to maintain your position and improve the body's alignment.

3. Squeezing the shoulders blades into each other will also help you firmly maintain the position for three to five breaths.

Coming out of the Asana

Lower the chin towards the chest, look in the direction of your toes and lower your hips towards the mat. Your partner follows suit.

THE IDEA GUIDING THE ASANA

You may not even touch your partner in this position, but the idea is to get into the asana by acknowledging each other's presence. The movements are graceful and appear visually beautiful. This asana also helps set the mood for practice. View this as another version of your 'namaste' to one another, in the middle of a sequence of postures.

AWARENESS

This asana makes you focus on the alignment of your body. While in the pose, mentally visualize your toes, ankles, knees, hips and shoulders being in a straight line. Picture all the muscles along the back of the body, from the heels to the shoulders, forming a strong supporting layer.

To maximize the benefits of this posture, focus on each intake of breath—after all, in this position the chest remains open.

ASANA 9:
TWISTING TWO POSE

PREPARATORY ASANA
Bharadvajasana (asana 1)

METHOD

Getting into the Asana

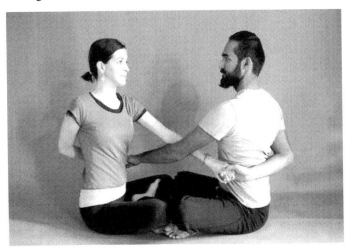

1. Sit facing each other in a cross-legged position, with your knees at the level of your partner's knees.
2. Look into each other's eyes and smile at one another.
3. Along with your partner, bend the right elbow and wrap the right arm around the back.

4. Extend the left arm forward and grab the right palm of the partner, while gently twisting the upper body. Your partner mirrors this.
5. Twist towards the right, looking over the left shoulder towards your partner. The partner mirrors this.
6. Roll the right shoulder back, and pull your partner's left arm with the bent right arm; again, the partner mirrors this.
7. You will feel your left arm getting pulled by the partner's right arm, and vice versa.

Maintaining the Asana

1. Look at your partner's face and see if s/he is comfortable with the push-and-pull of the asana and the adjustments you are making; re-adjust, if necessary.
2. Avoid any form of verbal communication and simply control the counterbalance offered while maintaining the asana. Try holding the pose for thirty seconds.

Coming out of the Asana

1. Come back to the centre.
2. Release the grip of each other's hands and relax.

THE IDEA GUIDING THE ASANA

There are three main ideas guiding this asana:

a) to twist the spine;
b) to provoke the mind by wrapping one arm around the body, and grabbing the partner's palm with the other hand;
c) to learn to cherish eye contact.

AWARENESS

Observe how your arms and hands cross your partner's in such a way that you lose all perception of which body part belongs to whom. Relish the way in which the arms link.

Soak in a chain reaction of movements, then enjoy your control over the asana.

Look into the eyes of your partner. Moreover, observe your chest lifting with each inhalation, and your shoulders rolling back with every exhalation.

ASANA 10:
FOLD INTO ME POSE

PREPARATORY ASANAS
Paschimottanasana (the variation under asana 2, padangusthasana)
Baddha konasana (asana 4)
Janu sirsasana (asana 22)

METHOD

Getting into the Asana

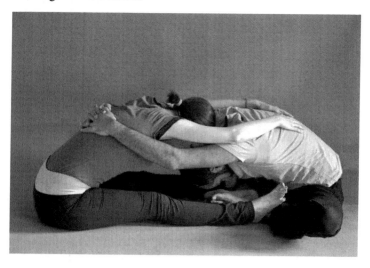

1. Your partner and you will sit in baddha konasana in front of each other.

2. Your partner extends her/his legs forward and places her/his feet on top of your shin bones.
3. Your partner and you will lift your arms up; then, one at a time—first you, and your partner after—bend forward and place your hands on each other's lower back. Your forehead rests on the mat and your partner bends forward in paschimottanasana, resting on your folded back. Your partner's posture, in turn, will help you fold further.

Maintaining the Asana

1. Your partner and you will continue gripping each other's lower back.
2. While following the sequence listed under 'getting into the asana', your partner will keep her/his legs straight and feet pushed into your shin bones to help you keep your heels close to the perineum while deepening the forward bend.
3. Keep breathing effortlessly, in conjunction with your partner, and hold the pose for about thirty seconds.

Coming out of the Asana

1. Your partner lifts her/his torso up, after 'maintaining the asana' (as described above).
2. This allows you to gently come out of the asana and relax.
3. Now, repeat this asana, flipping roles.

THE IDEA GUIDING THE ASANA

The idea guiding this asana is that both your partner and you give and receive support simultaneously while enjoying two different kinds of stretches.

If you're the one above: Your body, in paschimottanasana, gets support from the partner in baddha konasana. You enjoy a stretch that lengthens your spine.

If you're the one below: Your body, in baddha konasana, is challenged and your hips open.

AWARENESS

While surrendering to this position, both your partner and you will experience an overwhelming sense of humility; soak in the experience. Become familiar with the movement of your partner's breath, while staying in touch with the sound of your own respiration.

ASANA 11:
TWISTING INTO THE SIDE
BEND POSE

PREPARATORY ASANAS
Bharadvajasana (asana 1)
Ardha matsyendrasana (asana 21)

METHOD

Getting into the Asana: Stretch 1

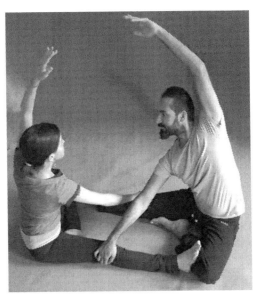

1. Sit cross-legged with your back straight and shoulders relaxed.
2. Make a fist out of your right hand and tuck it on the outer side of the left knee.
3. Raise your left arm straight and parallel to the floor.
4. Press the right fist against the left knee and twist the upper body towards the left, squeezing your left shoulder blade in and looking back over your left arm.
5. Bring your left arm down without changing the position of your upper body.
6. Place your left palm on the mat close to your hip.
7. Keep your left arm straight and continue to twist even further.
8. Release your hands after thirty seconds and return to a neutral position. Repeat the sequence with the other side.

Getting into the Asana: Stretch 2

1. Start, as with the previous asana, by sitting cross-legged with the back straight and shoulders relaxed.
2. Place your right hand on top of your left knee.
3. Lift your left arm up, with your torso slightly tilted towards the left knee and the spine straight.
4. Now begin tilting towards the right, offering a long stretch to the left side of your torso. The left arm remains straight and as close as possible to the ear.
5. Look towards the ceiling and make sure your torso is open and twisted—such that the sight of the ceiling is not covered by your left arm.
6. Keep breathing in the posture for about thirty seconds.
7. To come out of the position, simply release your left arm and bring your torso back to neutral. Repeat the sequence with the other side.

Getting into the Asana: What Follows

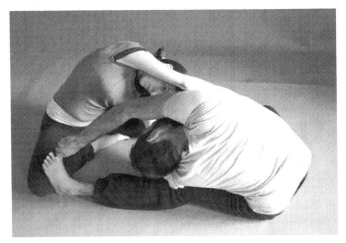

1. Sit in front of your partner. Extend your left leg out to the side, bending the right knee such that there is a 90-degree angle between your bent right leg and your outstretched left leg.

2. Your partner, who faces you, sits in the same position, so that the two of you mirror each other.

3. Your left foot touches your partner's right bent leg and vice versa.

4. Raise your right arm and tilt towards the left, moving the outstretched arm over the head until the right hand touches the toes of the left foot. Your partner mirrors this.

5. From this position, extend your left arm and reach out with this hand to the extended left leg of the partner in front. Your partner mirrors this, too.

6. Hook your left hand under the shoulder blade of your partner, even as your partner mirrors this.

7. Now each of you will gently pull your left arm towards yourself, and help the partner twist.

Maintaining the Asana

1. Keep your left arm hidden behind your ear to maintain the lateral stretch.
2. Keep the chest open towards the ceiling.
3. Breathe deeply into the body.
4. Maintain your grip on your partner's shoulder blade and help your partner twist and lengthen the spine at the same time.
5. Remind your partner to breathe.
6. Let your partner know if the stretch feels good.
7. Smile, even as you look into your partner's eyes. Hold this pose for thirty seconds.

Coming out of the Asana

1. Each of you releases the other's arm.
2. Each of you removes your foot from the other's knee.

THE IDEA GUIDING THE ASANA

This asana hopes to create a 'frame' with two bodies—an arrangement where every pull and push changes the kind of stretch each of you feels. This asana will also help both your partner and you understand each other's physical limits.

AWARENESS

Observe the composition of your two bodies—how they complement each other and form a rectangular frame on the yoga mat. Pay attention to each intake of breath. Experience the soothing touch of your partner. Become increasingly aware of how easy it is to keep your chest open and deepen the stretch, with the support and grip provided by a fellow practitioner.

ASANA 12:
TWO PIGEONS POSE

PREPARATORY ASANA
Rajakapotasana (asana 25)

METHOD

Getting into the Asana

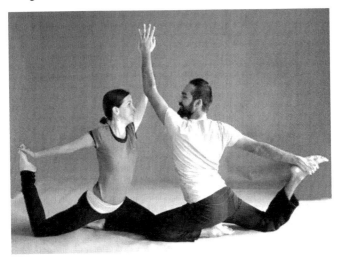

1. Get into rajakapotasana, with your partner facing and mirroring you.
2. Synchronize the extended legs, such that they are in one line.
3. Now, your partner and you will bend your respective right legs.

4. Grab your right ankle from the inside with your right hand, as your partner mirrors this.
5. Once you are holding your ankle (as is your partner), find your centre of balance. Now, carefully raise your left arm up, as your partner follows suit, and join your palm with your partner's.

Maintaining the Asana

1. Keep your palms firmly pressed against each other and ensure that your chest remains raised.
2. Keep breathing effortlessly.
3. Look into each other's eyes for about thirty seconds.

Coming out of the Asana

1 In conjunction with your partner, lower your hands down to the mat and press your palms into the mat.
2. Release the ankle that is at the back and straighten that leg out; your partner mirrors this move.
3. Both of you will roll to one side and come out of the position.

THE IDEA GUIDING THE ASANA

Rajakapotasana demands good balance, focus, strength and flexibility. In the 'partnering' format, you get to overcome some of these challenges as you place your palm against your partner's; this helps each of you give the other support. Though the 'two pigeons pose' might seem tricky at first, once you manage to enter a comfort zone, both of you will have fun maintaining your balance together.

This asana also gives your partner and you an opportunity to stretch the thigh muscles and open the chest.

Best of all, you get to break the ice, as both of you laugh while trying to maintain a kind of equilibrium.

AWARENESS

Observe the elevation offered to the chest with every inhalation and pay attention to the counterbalancing forces that keep your spine arched and your chest open. Observe how the lower back muscles get activated in order to maintain balance. Notice the smile on your partner's face once a kind of equilibrium is achieved.

ASANA 13:
TWIN POSE

PREPARATORY ASANAS
Shashankasana (asana 9)
Padmasana (asana 19)
Janu sirsasana (asana 22)

METHOD

Getting into the Asana

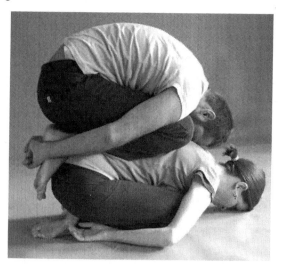

1. Your partner gets into shashankasana with her/his arms
    down, next to her/his body on the mat; your partner's palms

face towards the ceiling and her/his forehead gently rests on the mat.

2. Carefully place your hands on your partner's upper back and your knees on her/his lower back.

3. Maintaining your balance, fold into shashankasana on top of your partner's arched back.

Maintaining the Asana

1. Maintaining your balance in this asana is fun but it can also be challenging for both of you—one of you has to fold into a posture on the arched back of the other.

2. After following the sequence under 'getting into the asana', you remain stable by keeping your core active.

3. It's imperative for both of you to ensure that your breath flows normally, since this contributes to an overall sense of balance. Try maintaining the posture for about thirty seconds.

Coming out of the Asana

1. After following the sequence under 'getting into the asana' and 'maintaining the asana', when you need to come out of the posture, communicate with your partner. Gently lift your head up.

2. Your partner gently lifts her/his head up. S/he places her/his palms on the mat. After shifting her/his body weight towards her/his palms, your partner slowly stretches her/his legs, one by one.

3. You will now get to roll over to a parallel mat.

4. Repeat this asana, reversing roles.

THE IDEA GUIDING THE ASANA

This asana helps counter the backward bend of the previous asana (the 'two pigeons pose'). Shashankasana, in particular, is very restorative. It encourages your partner and you to surrender and relax, while supporting one another. It makes both of you feel like foetuses—as secure—and improves blood circulation.

AWARENESS

If you're the one above: Once you find a centre of balance, you will notice how soothing this posture can be—especially when you willingly take support from your partner below.

If you're the one below: You get to hear the sound of your partner's breath flowing in and out, close to your ear. Sense the gentle pressure you receive from her/his weight. Note how the balance of your partner above is linked to your own core strength and stability.

ASANA 14:
BLOOMING POSE

PREPARATORY ASANAS
Shashankasana (asana 9)
Bhujangasana (asana 10)
Natarajasana (asana 18)
Ardha matsyendrasana (asana 21)

METHOD

Getting into the Asana

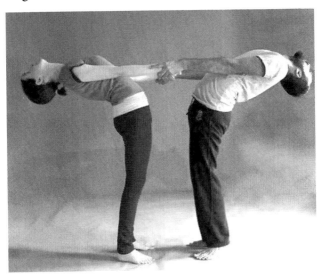

1. Stand in front of each other at arm's length.
2. Extend your arms, such that they are parallel to the floor. Your partner mirrors this. Hold your partner's wrists.
3. Lean back, looking into each other's eyes.
4. Your abdomen will push forward into your partner's, even as your partner mirrors this. Your backs will arch backwards.
5. Both of you will keep your arms straight. When your partner and you feel that the counterbalance offered by your respective body weights is granting both of you a sense of equilibrium, each of you will tilt your head backwards.

Maintaining the Asana

1. After following the sequence under 'getting into the asana', continue holding your partner's wrists, and counterbalance the weight of your body by pushing your abdomen forward. Your partner will, similarly, thrust her/his abdomen forward. Communicate with your partner to ensure that s/he is comfortable.
2. Both of you will keep your eyes open. Hold the pose for thirty seconds.

Coming out of the Asana

1. In conjunction with your partner, gently pull your abdomen back.
2. Bring your head to its original position by getting your chin close to your chest. This, in itself, will help you regain your balance. Your partner follows suit.
3. Both of you will come back to a neutral position, release your hands and relax.

THE IDEA GUIDING THE ASANA

This asana helps your partner and you recover a sense of balance; it also helps both of you to find new centres of equilibrium, as each acknowledges the body weight of the other. Your partner and you are offered a deep stretch with the backbend, and get to experience the mighty power of counterbalancing forces.

Besides, this pose inculcates the importance of mutual giving and receiving in a relationship.

AWARENESS

With this pose, you get to mirror your partner's feelings, as both of you get supported during the backbend, and slip deeper into an arch. Notice how you develop a new level of trust in your partner, as you bend backwards, relying on her/his support. Focus on your coordination with your partner—an absolute requirement for this asana—to reach the precise point where counterbalancing forces operate; now, two bodies will mutually support each other.

ASANA 15:
SIT TOGETHER POSE

PREPARATORY ASANA
Utkatasana (asana 8)

METHOD

Getting into the Asana

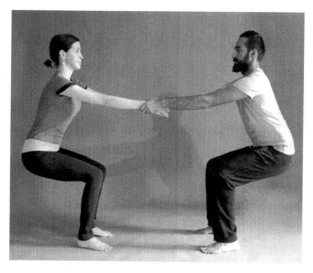

1. Stand tall with your feet parallel to those of your partner and face each other.
2. Hold your partner's hands.
3. Both of you will bend your legs very gently.

4. Your partner and you will straighten your arms and carefully 'pull back' while keeping your legs bent.
5. Both of you will lower your hips till they are in line with your knees; your thighs will be parallel to the floor. It will appear as though you are sitting on an imaginary chair.
6. Your partner and you can push your respective chests up and breathe.

Maintaining the Asana

1. After following the sequence under 'getting into the asana', your partner and you will keep the arms parallel to each other and continue sinking into the imaginary chair; this can be done when each of you gently pulls back by the arms, while keeping them linked.
2. The push-and-pull created by this asana will help both partners keep their spine straight.
3. Each of you will ensure that the thighs remain parallel to the floor and your feet firmly rooted in the mat. Hold the pose for about thirty seconds.

Coming out of the Asana

1. Straighten your legs and raise them up together.
2. Avoid straining your partner with your body's weight.
3. Release your hands in conjunction and relax.

THE IDEA GUIDING THE ASANA

This asana is a very good warm-up exercise that works on the thighs. Both of you will experience how core strength helps hold two bodies together.

Besides honing a sense of balance, this pose inculcates a feeling of trust in your partner.

AWARENESS

Focus on a sense of warmth rising from within the thighs. Notice how the push-and-pull of the arms allows two bodies to counterbalance one another, without any major effort. Make note of how crucial non-verbal communication and coordination with the partner are, if both of you are to maintain an even distribution of weight and hold your balance.

ASANA 16:
LONDON BRIDGE POSE

PREPARATORY ASANAS
Padangusthasana (asana 2)
Adho mukha svanasana or parvatasana (asana 12)
Utthita trikonasana (asana 15)

METHOD

Getting into the Asana

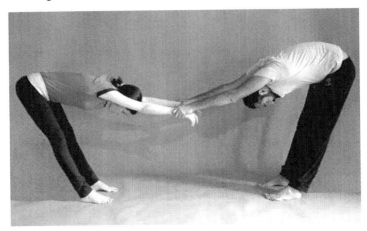

1. Maintain the hand lock of the previous asana ('sit together pose').
2. From here, get the legs straight and point your hips back, bending the back forward. Your partner keeps pace.

3. Keep holding your partner from the wrist and pull each other's arms by shifting the body weight towards the tailbone.
4. Keep your spine as straight as possible and in line with your arms and the arms of your partner.

Maintaining the Asana

1. After following the sequence under 'getting into the asana', continue holding your partner's wrists tightly.
2. Avoid straining your partner with your body weight (and ensure that your partner avoids doing this, too); this will allow both of you to lengthen the spine.
3. Keep your tailbone pointing outwards and your legs straight, in conjunction with your partner.
4. Breathe deeply with your partner and hold the pose for a minute.

Coming out of the Asana

1. Breathe in and make eye contact with your partner.
2. Bend your knees very gently and pull your chest back, in conjunction with your partner.
3. Slowly rise up together; your spine will be parallel to your partner's.
4. Release your hands and breathe comfortably.

THE IDEA GUIDING THE ASANA

This asana works at the physical level by stretching the hamstrings and lengthening the back. It helps both your partner and you distribute your weight evenly and appreciate the counterbalancing forces at work.

At an emotional and psychological level, this pose helps build trust between the two of you.

AWARENESS

Observe how directing the body's weight towards the pulled-in kneecaps grants the hamstrings a thorough stretch.

Also appreciate the trust your partner has in you when s/he lets go and relies on you to maintain balance, as much as you rely on her/him.

ASANA 17:
LONDON BRIDGE II POSE

PREPARATORY ASANA
Adho mukha svanasana or parvatasana (asana 12)

METHOD

Getting into the Asana

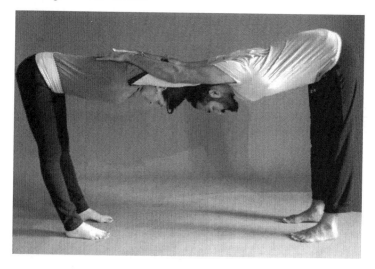

1. Begin by standing at arm's length from each other.
2. Place your hands on each other's shoulder blades and bend
   forward. As the body sinks, the hands slide further down
   towards the shoulder blades.

3. Gently step back and start pressing your hands on the back of your partner. Your partner mirrors this.
4. Get the arms in line with each other and the spine.
5. Your partner and you will breathe, keeping the neck loose.

Maintaining the Asana

1. Your partner and you hold the asana by continuing to press your hands on each other's shoulders.
2. Breathe deeply and encourage your partner to respire. Try holding the asana for about a minute.

Coming out of the Asana

1. Breathe in, lift your head up and pull your chest up. Your partner will mirror this.
2. Your body will come out of the asana effortlessly.

THE IDEA GUIDING THE ASANA

This asana helps open the chest and the shoulders, so blood circulates towards the upper part of the body. This pose also lengthens the spine and soothes the lower back. This is an excellent exercise if your partner and you wish to explore the counterbalancing effects of partner yoga.

AWARENESS

Tune into the touch of your partner's hands on your shoulders, and your own grip on your partner's shoulders.

Notice how your breath becomes slow and goes deep. Pay attention to the sound of your breath and your partner's as you support each other with the forward bend.

Enjoy the stretch offered to the back. Compare how the stretch and the balance offered by this asana differ from those of the previous asana ('London bridge pose').

ASANA 18:
TREE OF FRIENDSHIP POSE

PREPARATORY ASANAS
Garudasana (asana 13)
Vrikshasana (asana 24)

METHOD

Getting into the Asana

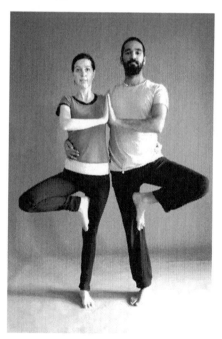

1. Stand next to your partner with your feet parallel to each other in one straight line.
2. Gently place your left foot on the inside of your right thigh.
3. Your partner places her/his right foot on the inside of her/his left thigh.
4. Let the side of your hips touch your partner's hip. Wrap your inner arm around your partner's waist, while your partner mirrors this gesture.
5. Your outer arm and that of your partner are bent towards the front, with the hands touching each other, in the prayer position.

Maintaining the Asana

1. Both partners help each other maintain balance.
2. Press your palms firmly together, which allows the asana to gain in strength.
3. Breathe in and out gently, matching your partner's inhalations and exhalations. Try holding the pose for about eight rounds of inhaling and exhaling.

Coming out of the Asana

1. Your partner and you will lower your legs and simply come out of the asana.
2. Keep holding your partner while s/he is standing.

THE IDEA GUIDING THE ASANA

With vrikshasana in the partner yoga format, a sense of balance comes more easily; both partners support each other by staying upright and by pressing their palms together. This grants the posture stability.

AWARENESS

Your partner and you should be conscious of all those parts of the body that are in contact—especially focusing on the link between the two hands in a prayer position, and the gentle pressure that the partner's body weight exerts on your hand. Also, become aware of the position of your foot on the mat, and the role this plays in rooting you to the ground, as though you're a tree—granting you a sense of balance.

Focus your gaze on a point in front of you (a wall or any object), at eye level or a little higher, to help keep your body still, straight and poised, and to facilitate your partner's ability to maintain balance. Your partner should follow this instruction, too.

Experience the feelings of proximity and mutual support that the 'tree of friendship pose' fosters.

ASANA 19:
LET'S FOLD AND HOLD POSE

PREPARATORY ASANAS
Padangusthasana (asana 2)
Padmasana (asana 19)
Janu sirsasana (asana 22)

METHOD

Getting into the Asana

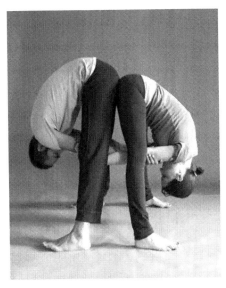

1. Your partner and you stand back-to-back, maintaining space between your two bodies.

2. Raise your arms and bend forward to touch your toes; your partner mirrors this.

3. Now, extend your arms and grab the shoulders of your partner, pulling her/him towards you; your partner mirrors this. This will help both of you deepen the forward bend.

Maintaining the Asana

1. Grab the shoulders of your partner firmly.
2. Keep your head and your neck relaxed.
3. Keep your legs completely straight.
4. Breathe comfortably for thirty seconds.

Coming out of the Asana

1. Release your partner's shoulders and drop your arms. Your partner follows suit.
2. Both of you can now slowly uncurl, vertebra by vertebra, keeping the head relaxed. Roll out of the position, with the head coming up last.

THE IDEA GUIDING THE ASANA

This asana helps both of you stretch the hamstrings and deepen the forward bend in an enjoyable way. You (along with your partner) also get to work on your balance by distributing your body weight towards your toes, while leaning against a fellow practitioner's body.

To enjoy the assistance provided by your partner, work on grabbing her/his shoulders, which allows you to deepen the fold.

AWARENESS

Observe the parts of your body that are in touch with your partner. Also, make note of the weight and pressure exerted on you by your partner's body as s/he bends forward and pushes against your waist. Observe how, while counterbalancing one another, the two of you manage to support each other and maintain the posture. Remain conscious of your breath, and your partner's, as both of you inhale and exhale deeply while stretching.

You can sense the weight of your head, as it hangs loose, when you fold your body such that you elongate your spine; your partner is granted this sensation, too. Besides, you'll perceive the hamstrings stretching when your partner grabs you by the shoulders and makes you bend forward and move still deeper into the pose; again, this sensation can be experienced by your fellow practitioner.

ASANA 20:
CARRY ME POSE

PREPARATORY ASANAS
Bhujangasana (asana 10)
Natarajasana (asana 18)
Halasana (asana 20)

METHOD

Getting into the Asana

1. Stand back-to-back with each other.
2. Your partner and you will now move your arms to the level of your shoulders.
3. 'Wear' the arms of your partner as though they are the straps of a bag.
4. Match the arch of your back with the arch of your partner's back.

Maintaining the Asana

1. After following the sequence under 'getting into the asana', while lifting your partner up, make sure your legs are straight and hips pushed out to match the arch of your partner's back. You can create a 'safety belt' by moving your arms behind and wrapping them around your partner's back.
2. Your partner will completely let go and relax, evenly distributing her/his body weight on your back. Your partner will keep her/his arms over your belly or head. S/he could, if flexible, reach out for her/his feet. Together, you could try holding the pose for thirty seconds.

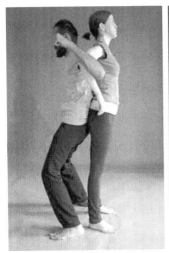
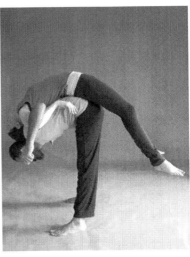
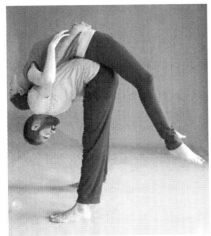
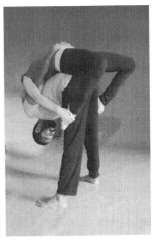

Coming out of the Asana

1. After following the sequence under 'getting into the asana' and 'maintaining the asana', slowly bend your knees and lift your torso up, ensuring that the belt of the arms is maintained till your partner's feet are down on the mat.
2. Release the lock of the hands while still keeping your arms under the arms of your partner.
3. Because of the sudden flow of blood on descent, the partner might feel a bit dizzy. So make sure your partner has regained her/his balance and is standing comfortably on her/his feet, before letting go.
4. Reverse roles and repeat the asana.

THE IDEA GUIDING THE ASANA

Achieving the right equilibrium—such that both of you are comfortable practising your respective parts of the asana—can be challenging. But this posture helps your partner and you find your centre of balance; besides, it lets you explore the body's reaction to and interaction with another person's movements.

Through this asana, both of you learn to lean on one another physically and mentally, and build a foundation of trust.

If you're the one above/being carried: The aim is to deepen the arch of your back and open the chest to facilitate the intake of breath. Besides, this pose helps you build your confidence in your partner—you need to reach a point where you're happy to be lifted, while the eyes remain closed, and your mind relaxed, knowing that your partner will take good care of you.

If you're the one below/carrying: This pose provides a great stretch to your hamstrings, as you bend forward.

AWARENESS

Observe how your partner and you have managed to synchronize movements, and have counterbalanced one another. Make note of the shape and contour of your back against your partner's, and feel the bond between the two of you grow both physically and mentally.

If you're the one above/being carried: Observe your body as it lets go, certain that your partner will take care of its safety; soak in an overwhelming sense of liberation.

If you're the one below/carrying: As you offer support, you'll sense your confidence growing; notice how empowering this is. Also remain conscious of the fact that your faith in your partner keeps increasing, as you learn that s/he will not jeopardize your sense of balance.

ASANA 21:
ULTIMATE T POSE

PREPARATORY ASANAS
Setu bandhasana (asana 6)
Shashankasana (asana 9)
Adho mukha svanasana or parvatasana (asana 12)
Garudasana (asana 13)

METHOD

Getting into the Asana

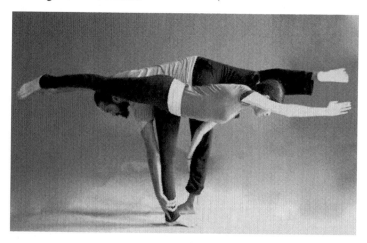

1. Get into tadasana—a pose where you stand with your legs
    together. Raise your arms straight up. Your partner follows
    suit.

2. Place yourself shoulder-to-shoulder with your partner, such that the two of you face opposite directions.

3. Lean your outer leg back, launch it off the mat, and start bending forward with the torso, keeping your arms extended. Keep raising your outer leg further up and lower the torso down until the arms, torso and the outstretched leg are in a straight line. Your partner will mirror this sequence.

Maintaining the Asana

1. Bring your inner arm down and grab your partner's inner leg. Ensure that the arms, torso and the outstretched leg are still in a straight line and parallel to the floor. Keep your eyes open.

2. Keep a firm grip on your partner's leg, so the weight of your body is counterbalanced, and you remain stable.

3. Your partner mirrors this sequence, and together, you hold the pose for about thirty seconds.

Coming out of the Asana

1. Release the grip of your hand, and place the lifted leg down on the mat. Your partner does this in conjunction with you.

2. Along with your partner, come back to a vertical position, with your arms down.

THE IDEA GUIDING THE ASANA

With this asana, both of you feel your hamstrings stretch and get to strengthen your lower and upper back muscles. Without being wholly aware, you end up granting support to one another, and increasing the posture's stability. This asana helps you experience, at a physical level, the give and take any relationship asks for.

AWARENESS

Focus on bringing your torso and your lifted leg parallel to the floor, and parallel to the body of your partner. Your partner makes a similar attempt. Visualize the joint asana as the capital letter 'T'. Breathe calmly and, in conjunction with your partner, attend to the foot that roots you to the ground.

This asana activates every practitioner's proprioception skills, as you cannot really see whether your leg is at the same level as your arm, and whether your limbs are at the same plane as your partner's.

ASANA 22:
BACKPACK POSE

PREPARATORY ASANAS
Matsyasana (asana 16)
Natarajasana (asana 18)
Halasana (asana 20)

METHOD

Getting into the Asana

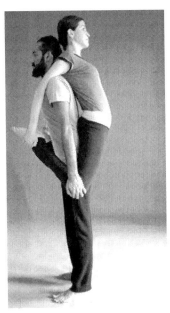

1. Bend forward (you can bend your knees ever so slightly).
2. Your partner arches her/his back on your back.
3. 'Wear' the arms of your partner as though they are the straps of a bag.
4. Lean forward and take your partner on your back.
5. Stretch your arms back and grab your partner's knees.
6. Wait for your partner to grab her/his own ankles.
7. Once your partner has gripped her/his ankles, gently lift yourself up, so that your spine is straight, and support your partner by keeping your hands under her/his knees.

Maintaining the Asana

1. While following the sequence under 'getting into the asana' and carrying your partner, ensure that your body weight shifts to the front. This will provide greater comfort to your back and make it relatively easier to maintain balance. Your partner, too, will be able to lean against your body with ease.
2. Once your partner and you feel comfortable and confident in the posture, start taking a few steps—as though you are a tourist backpacking! This is bound to induce laughter, and make this among the most enjoyable partner yoga asanas!

Coming out of the Asana

1. Communicate with your partner when you are carrying her/him, after 'getting into the asana' and 'maintaining the asana' as previously described. Lean forward slightly—enough to shift the weight of your body to your back.
2. Encourage your partner let go of her/his ankles and slowly place her/his feet on the mat.
3. Reverse roles and repeat the asana.

THE IDEA GUIDING THE ASANA

This is an entertaining pose.

If you're lifting your partner: This pose allows you to carry her/him such that her/his weight on your back does not cause any strain—just as a backpack causes little discomfort.

If you're being carried: This posture offers a good backbend; it works on deepening the arch of your back.

AWARENESS

If you're lifting your partner: Notice the way the underarms of your partner settle on top of your shoulder, as s/he is being carried. Also, note that the support you offer your partner under her/his knees feels comfortable for both of you, for the giver and the receiver.

If you're being carried: While the partner above may, to some extent, perceive the weight of your body, you get to soak in a sense of support/comfort, and a feeling of completion as your body is kept in place.

ASANA 23:
TWO MOUNTAINS POSE

PREPARATORY ASANAS
Naukasana (asana 3)
Adho mukha svanasana or parvatasana (asana 12)
Garudasana (asana 13)
Matsyasana (asana 16)
Ardha matsyendrasana (asana 21)

METHOD

Getting into the Asana

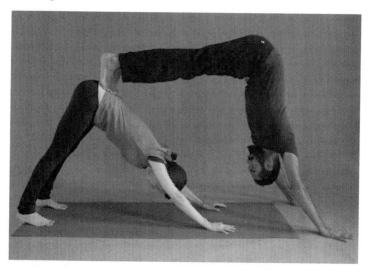

1. Your partner gets down on the mat into adho mukha svanasana or parvatasana.
2. Now, it's time for you to bend forward and place your hands on the mat, in front of, and in line with, your partner's hands.
3. Lift your right foot and gently place it on your partner's back while s/he holds her body in adho mukha svanasana or parvatasana.
4. Gently push your partner's lower back away by keeping your right leg straight and parallel to the floor. Now, bring your left leg up, while maintaining your balance. Place your left foot on your partner's back, and next to your right foot. Both your feet, therefore, will be on your partner's back and your legs will be straight.
5. Your partner continues holding the original pose of adho mukha svanasana or parvatasana; the pressure of your body on her/his back will help your partner push her/his heels into the mat.

Maintaining the Asana

1. While following the sequence under 'getting into the asana', you'll keep your tailbone pointed towards the ceiling for better control over your body.
2. As for your partner, s/he'll settle into adho mukha svanasana or parvatasana; the push of your feet will help your partner lengthen her/his back even further. Together, you can attempt holding the pose for about thirty seconds.

Coming out of the Asana

1. Very gently, after following the sequence under 'getting into the asana' and 'maintaining the asana', lower your right leg and place it on the mat; the left leg follows.
2. Your partner follows the instructions for 'coming out of the asana' under asana 12 of 'the preparatory series', to ease out

of adho mukha svanasana or parvatasana.
3.   Now, repeat this asana, reversing roles.

THE IDEA GUIDING THE ASANA

This asana is meant to offer both your partner and you a 'stretch' to the legs and back.

AWARENESS

Observe how both you and your partner have your arms parallel to each other.

If you are the one below: Pay attention to the fact that when your partner on top pushes against your lower back, it helps your heels settle onto the mat. While maintaining your position, if you can lift your head up and look into the eyes of your partner, you'll experience the joys of non-verbal communication.

If you're the one above: Make note of your fingers spread out on the mat, or close to it; notice the strength of your arms in this posture. Observe how your body weight is distributed between your hands and legs.

ASANA 24:
SCORPION ON THE ROCK POSE

PREPARATORY ASANAS
Bharadvajasana (asana 1)
Padangusthasana (asana 2)
Ustrasana (asana 7)
Bhujangasana (asana 10)
Adho mukha svanasana or parvatasana (asana 12)
Natarajasana (asana 18)

METHOD

Getting into the Asana

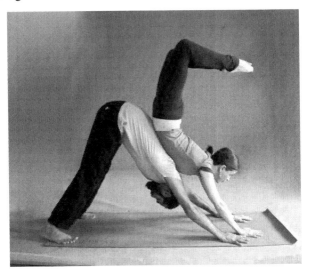

1. Get into adho mukha svanasana or parvatasana.
2. Your partner gently places her/his hands right next to your hands. Using your body as a lever, s/he hoists her/his body up, placing the knees on your lower back.
3. Your partner bends her/his legs and comfortably lowers the abdomen towards your back.
4. You will firmly hold your position in adho mukha svanasana or parvatasana, while your partner bends the legs and brings the toes towards her/his head.

Maintaining the Asana

1. While following the sequence under 'getting into the asana', your partner receives support from her/his hands and from your body.
2. Settle your heels on the mat and allow your chest to sink towards it to accommodate the partner above.
3. Your partner and you must slow your breaths and hold the pose for approximately thirty seconds.

Coming out of the Asana

1. After following the sequence under 'getting into the asana' and 'maintaining the asana', bend your knees and gently place them on the mat; your partner remains on your back.
2. Now, your partner stretches her/his legs towards the mat, and places her/his toes on its surface; using the hands for support, s/he comes out of the posture.
3. Relax. Then, reverse roles and repeat the asana.

THE IDEA GUIDING THE ASANA

This pose will allow your partner and you to take adho mukha svanasana or parvatasana to a whole new level.

If you're the one below: As you remain in adho mukha svanasana or parvatasana, your hamstrings get stretched.

If you're the one above: Your body is in bhujangasana. As you maintain the pose, the arch of your back deepens.

AWARENESS

Both your partner and you will pay attention to those body parts that are in contact. Both of you will also focus on your sense of balance, so as to strengthen it.

If you're the one below: Enjoy the feeling of the hamstrings stretching. Make note of your heels settling down on the mat, thanks to the weight of the partner on your back.

If you're the one above: Notice how your partner's back works as a lever against which you can lift your legs up in the air. Also notice your lower back muscles getting activated when you bend your knees and bring your toes towards the back of your head. Observe how the more you push into your partner's body, the more you manage to arch and lift your legs up. Don't forget noticing your palms and your fingers spread out on the mat! Feel your arms stretch and sense the support that your partner's body provides you.

ASANA 25:
THE WHEEL OF TWO POSE

PREPARATORY ASANAS
Setu bandhasana (asana 6)
Shashankasana (asana 9)
Adho mukha svanasana or parvatasana (asana 12)

METHOD

Getting into the Asana

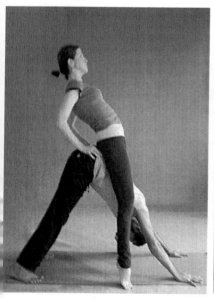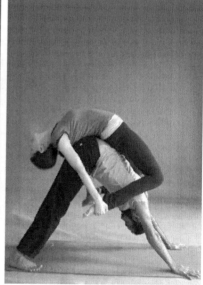

1. Hold adho mukha svanasana or parvatasana steadily, with a firm grip on the mat.
2. Your partner stands close to your hands with her/his legs wide, looking away from you.
3. Your partner leans back, and taking the support of your back, rests her/his hips on your lower back.
4. Your partner places her/his arms over her/his head and balances on your back.
5. S/he lifts the feet off the mat and bends the knees to grab her/his own ankles. Her body maintains a version of setu bandhasana.

Maintaining the Asana

1. After following the sequence under 'getting into the asana', your partner rests her/his head on the back of your thighs.
2. On your part, you will raise your tailbone to deepen the arch of your partner's back. Together, you can try holding the pose for thirty seconds.

Coming out of the Asana

1. After following the sequence under 'getting into the asana' and 'maintaining the asana', your partner releases her/his ankles gently and places her/his feet on the mat.
2. Using the strength of the core muscles, your partner straightens the spine and stands erect. Then, s/he settles the body into shashankasana.
3. Now, you are free to lower your knees to the mat and also settle into shashankasana.

THE IDEA GUIDING THE ASANA

In this asana, it looks as though the partner below is lifting the other one up and carrying all the weight. However, the fact is that both of you are 'receivers'—with the partner below holding a stable adho mukha svanasana or parvatasana pose thanks to the pressure of the partner above; and the partner above getting the support of the back of the one below.

This pose will also help your partner and you explore two classic yogic asanas—adho mukha svanasana or parvatasana and setu bandhasana—in a light-hearted, yet challenging way, with the elements of balance and mutual support introduced.

AWARENESS

Focus on the points of contact between your partner's body and your own; observe how two beings complement each other. Also, observe the way in which the weight of two bodies is distributed, helping both your partner and you experience more than what individual asanas could offer. Become aware of your partner's breath and your own, while maintaining the pose.

If you're the one below: Observe how the body weight of your partner above deeply roots you in adho mukha svanasana or parvatasana—your back is lengthened, your heels touch the mat and your hamstrings stretch.

If you're the one above: Observe how arching your body and using your partner's back for support while hoisting yourself off the mat, increases the backbend and makes the pose more entertaining!

ASANA 26:
DEFYING GRAVITY POSE

PREPARATORY ASANAS
Padangusthasana (asana 2)
Adho mukha svanasana or parvatasana (asana 12)
Chaturanga dandasana (asana 17)

METHOD

Getting into the Asana

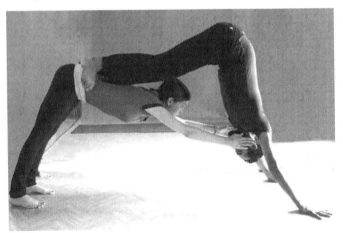

1. Let your partner get into a firm adho mukha svanasana or parvatasana pose.
2. Stand just beyond the hands of your partner and turn your back to her/him.

3. Bend forward and place your hands down on the mat, bending your knees slightly, if required.
4. Maintaining a firm grip on the mat, lift your right leg up and gently place your right foot on the lower back of your partner in adho mukha svanasana or parvatasana.
5. Once you're comfortably balanced, gently place your left foot next to the right foot on your partner's lower back.
6. To ensure that your partner is comfortable with the pressure you are exerting on her/his back, ask for feedback while placing your feet. Make sure you gently adjust your position so both of you feel stable and comfortable.
7. Firmly push your palms further into the mat and, with your legs straight and parallel to the floor, gently push the lower back of your partner further away.
8. Continue to push gently until your partner feels as though s/he is being lifted up. Once s/he feels adequately supported, s/he will be able to lift her/his hands off the mat.

Maintaining the Asana

1. While following the sequence under 'getting into the asana', your partner keeps her/his legs straight, the hands off the mat and leans forward while her/his torso remains lifted up.
2. Your partner's arms remain straight and in line with the spine.
3. Ensure that your legs remain firmly pushed against the lower back of your partner, and exploit your body weight to keep your partner's hands off the mat. Try holding the pose for thirty seconds.

Coming out of the Asana

1. After following the sequence under 'getting into the asana', and 'maintaining the asana', gently decrease the pressure on

your partner's back and allow her/him to settle her/his hands on the mat.

2. Lower your right foot to the mat and, maintaining your balance, bring the other foot down as well. Stand up.

3. Reverse roles and repeat the asana.

THE IDEA GUIDING THE ASANA

This is an exciting asana, since your partner and you get to arrange yourselves in precisely the direction where force is applied, while maintaining your balance.

AWARENESS

If you're the one with your feet off the mat: Focus your attention on the point of contact between your feet and your partner's lower back, while pushing against your partner. Notice how effortlessly the final position is achieved as a result of the application of the right amount of force in the right direction.

If you're the one in adho mukha svanasana or parvatasana: Enjoy the stretch offered to your back. Remain tuned in to the sensation of touch (as your partner's feet push against your lower back) and notice any increase in pressure. Note the shift in your body weight towards your heels as the result of your partner's push.

ASANA 27:
THE FROG AND FISH POSE

PREPARATORY ASANAS
Adho mukha svanasana or parvatasana (asana 12)
Matsyasana (asana 16)

METHOD

Getting into the Asana

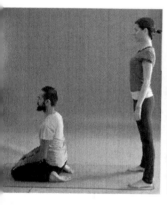 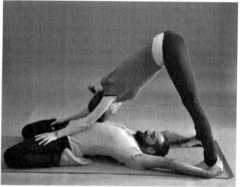

1. Sit on your heels. Gently place your elbows back and lower the upper back to the mat, so you're in matsyasana.
2. Your partner stands close to your head with her/his feet as wide as your shoulders are.
3. From here, your partner bends forward and gets into adho

mukha svanasana or parvatasana by placing her/his hands on your lower thighs/knees.

4. Continue to lie down on the mat, reach out and grab your partner's ankles.

Maintaining the Asana

1. After following the sequence under 'getting into the asana', keep looking into your partner's eyes.
2. Your partner pushes her/his heels into the mat to stretch and lengthen the back.
3. Your partner also continues to keep her/his arms extended, pressing your thighs/knees with her/his palms.
4. Both partners continue to breathe normally, while holding the asana for a minute.

Coming out of the Asana

1. After following the sequence under 'getting into the asana' and 'maintaining the asana', release your partner's ankles while s/he walks back with her/his hands, until balance is regained.
2. Reverse roles, and attempt the asana again.

THE IDEA GUIDING THE ASANA

If you're the one below: This pose aims to stretch your thighs without arching your back.

If you're the one above: This asana hopes to exploit your body weight as you remain in adho mukha svanasana or parvatasana.

AWARENESS

If you're the one below: Make note of the stretch along your thighs, as you hold your partner's ankles. Also observe how the pressure your partner applies with her/his hands allows you to keep your thighs pressed against the mat—this makes you stretch without overarching the back.

If you're the one above: The fact that your partner holds your ankles makes adho mukha svanasana or parvatasana feel stable and secure. It allows you to lengthen your spine and sink deep into the posture. Enjoy the stretch offered to the front of your thighs.

ASANA 28:
SUSPENDED ME POSE

PREPARATORY ASANAS
Utkatasana (asana 8)
Utthita trikonasana (asana 15)
Natarajasana, (asana 18)
Janu sirsasana (asana 22)

METHOD

Getting into the Asana

1. Lie down on the mat and raise your legs. Your partner stands in front of you, facing you, with her/his feet slightly apart.
2. Bend your knees and place your feet just below your partner's hip girdle.
3. Reach out with your arms and hold the hands of your partner, who leans forward.
4. Pull your partner with your hands and push her/him with your legs—till such time that your legs are straight and your partner has her/his feet off the mat.
5. Communicate with your partner and see if s/he is comfortable.
6. While maintaining your partner's balance and your own, ask your partner to join her/his hands together, at the back of her/his head, as though praying.
7. Hold your partner's elbows and push your arms so they are straight.

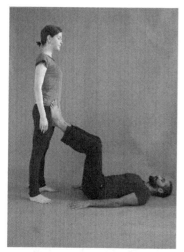
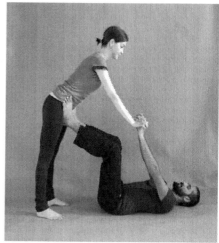
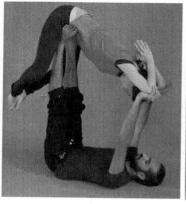
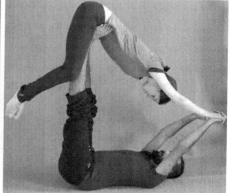

Maintaining the Asana

1. After following the sequence under 'getting into the asana', keep
    your arms straight, so the elbows of the partner above you
    remain pushed; this will help your partner relax her/his neck.

2. Your partner above keeps the soles of her/his feet joined and knees apart, so as to distribute her/his weight properly. This will make it relatively easier for you to balance her/his body. Your partner and you can try maintaining the pose for about thirty seconds.

Coming out of the Asana

1. After following the sequence under 'getting into the asana' and 'maintaining the asana', hold the arms of your partner, and bend your legs till the feet of your partner touch the mat. Ensure that your partner is standing and well-balanced.
2. Reverse roles and repeat the asana.

THE IDEA GUIDING THE ASANA

If you're the one below: This pose helps strengthen your spine and lengthen your arms.

If you're the one above: This asana—by tapping into the forces of gravity and offering your back a good stretch—helps you relax.

AWARENESS

If you're the one below: Pay attention to the way in which your partner's body balances itself on your feet, and the variations in the distribution of her/his body weight with every movement.

If you're the one above: Make note of the gentle weight of your head and how your spine gets aligned in this position. Pay attention to how the force of gravity, the support of your partner's feet and your own inverted position offer a definite 'stretch' to your spine, lengthening it. Besides, focus on the stretch offered to your triceps and the gentle yet firm push of your partner against your elbows—which help open your chest. Enjoy the sensations of well-being and relaxation; let go of all anxieties.

ASANA 29:
FLYING YOGI POSE

PREPARATORY ASANAS
Padangusthasana (asana 2)
Dhanurasana (asana 5)
Adho mukha svanasana or parvatasana (asana 12)
Chaturanga dandasana (asana 17)
Halasana (asana 20)
Janu sirsasana (asana 22)

METHOD

Getting into the Asana

1. Lie down on your back on the mat and lift both your legs such that they are at a 90-degree angle with the floor. Your arms are straight and alongside your body, and your palms are facing down.
2. Your partner stands near your feet, facing you.
3. Bend your legs in order to place your feet on the lower abdomen of your partner, close to her/his hipbone area.
4. Your partner slowly bends forward and, arms extended, reaches out to grip your hands.
5. Once you feel that the arms of your partner are secure and her/his feet are supporting her/his body weight, extend both your legs out, lifting your partner off the mat.
6. Your partner will keep her/his body supple. If flexible, s/he can get into dhanurasana, by reaching out for her/his feet with the hands, while balancing on your feet.

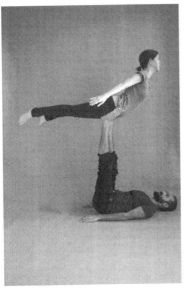 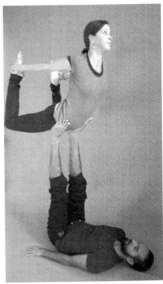

Maintaining the Asana

1. After following the sequence under 'getting into the asana', keep looking at your partner.

2. Your partner maintains a backward bend—this is done by putting the upper and lower back muscles as also the buttocks to work. Try holding the pose for thirty seconds.

Coming out of the Asana

1. After following the sequence under 'getting into the asana' and 'maintaining the asana', communicate with your partner. Tell her/him to lower the hands and soften the back, which will allow her/him to lower the body down.

2. Once your partner is close to you, reach out with your arms and hold her/his hands; gently bring her/him to the mat.

3. Reverse roles and repeat the pose.

THE IDEA GUIDING THE ASANA

This asana requires both partners to communicate. Where one experiences the joys of trusting, the other gets to build her/his self-confidence.

If you're the one below: You need to have faith in your abilities and hold your partner such that s/he is stable and comfortable.

If you're the one above: You need to have confidence in your partner to stretch your body out without any extra support—that is, apart from the touch of your partner's feet around the hip area.

AWARENESS

Both your partner and you need to focus on your breath as you maintain your balance in the asana.

If you're the one below: Focus on the point of contact between the soles of your feet and your partner's body, and notice how the body weight of your partner gets distributed.

If you're the one above: Make note of the moment when you feel sufficiently supported and entirely in control of your balance, such that you can raise your torso and stretch out your entire body. Pay attention to the activation of the muscles of your lower back as you rise up, open your arms out and then get into dhanurasana.

ASANA 30:
FLYING BOW POSE

PREPARATORY ASANAS
Dhanurasana (asana 5)
Setu bandhasana (asana 6)

METHOD

Getting into the Asana

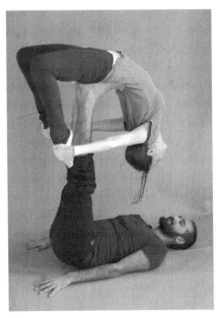

1. Lie down on your back on the mat.
2. Lift your legs up at a 90-degree angle.
3. Your partner stands close to your feet, facing away from you.
4. Your partner gently arches her/his back and leans against your feet.
5. Bend your knees a little, taking the weight of your partner and allowing your partner to arch the back still deeper.
6. Lay your hands on the shoulders of your partner. Lift and push your legs into the lower back of your partner, until your legs are straight.
7. Your partner lifts her/his feet off the mat.
8. Hold your partner's shoulders and guide her/him such that your partner can grab her/his ankles, and get into dhanurasana. Then place your hands on the mat, the palms facing down.

Maintaining the Asana

1. After following the sequence under 'getting into the asana', keep your feet firmly on your partner's back and make sure that your partner is comfortable with the arch in her/his back.
2. Your partner holds her/his ankles and keeps the head relaxed; exploiting the expansion this offers the ribcage and the chest, s/he inhales as deeply as possible.
3. Your partner keeps her/his body weight divided between her/his feet and shoulders. Once the partner is comfortable, s/he may release the legs, so s/he is suspended and parallel to the floor; s/he'll also release the hands and grab your head. Both your partner and you can try holding this pose for thirty seconds.

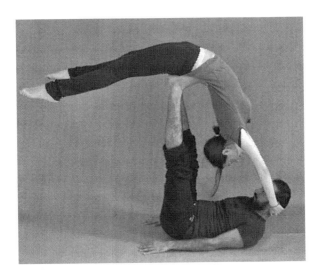

Coming out of the Asana

1. After following the sequence under 'getting into the asana' and 'maintaining the asana', place your hands firmly on the shoulders of your partner.
2. Your partner communicates with you and releases her/his ankles gently. S/he keeps the head relaxed.
3. Very gently, bend your knees and allow your partner to lower her/his feet on the mat.
4. Your partner uses her/his core strength to regain balance.
5. Reverse roles and repeat the asana.

THE IDEA GUIDING THE ASANA

This is a pose that promotes trust between two practitioners.

If you're the one below: This pose does wonders to your self-confidence as you seemingly balance your partner on your feet!

If you're the one above: This pose takes dhanurasana to a whole new level and as you slip into it, you feel the effects of gravity. Besides helping you experience a different kind of balancing asana—one that comes with an inversion—this pose opens the chest and promotes inhalation.

AWARENESS

Both your partner and you should remain conscious of each breath and observe how it helps establish a connection. Each of you should focus on the touch of the other—whether the point of contact is the feet or the hands—and make note of how this provides the support you need to maintain the posture.

If you're the one below: Observe how the alignment of your legs and hands on your partner's shoulders grants her/him a sense of balance. Note how this gives you a sense of steadiness, too.

If you're the one above: Make yourself comfortable in a suspended backbend. Enjoy the inversion with confidence, even while remaining conscious of the kind of support your partner offers.

ASANA 31:
UP IN THE CLOUDS POSE

PREPARATORY ASANAS
Dhanurasana (asana 5)
Ustrasana (asana 7)
Chaturanga dandasana (asana 17)

METHOD

Getting into the Asana

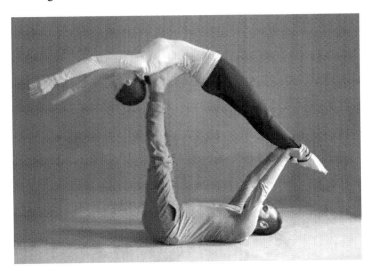

1. Lie down on the mat.
2. Your partner stands, facing you, with her/his feet on either side of your torso.

3. Now, lift your legs up at a 90-degree angle; your feet remain flexed.

4. Your partner slowly arches rearwards until the middle of her/his back comes into contact with your feet.

5. Bend your knees slightly so that you can adjust the position of your feet on your partner's back; this helps your partner arch more effectively.

6. Grab your partner's ankles and gently lift her/his feet off the mat, one by one, as s/he can sink deep into a backbend.

7. Your partner stretches the arms over the head to shift the weight of her/his body; this will not only help your partner maintain balance but will also grant her/him a graceful arch.

Maintaining the Asana

1. After completing the sequence under 'getting into the asana', keep your eyes open to remain oriented. Avoid bending the knees to maintain balance. The legs can be kept at a little over 90 degrees to balance your partner's body weight.

2. Your partner keeps her/his arms straight to maintain balance, and ensures that her/his back remains arched. Your partner and you can try holding the pose for thirty seconds.

Coming out of the Asana

1. After completing the sequence under 'getting into the asana' and 'maintaining the asana', your partner brings her/his arms to the sides of the body.

2. S/he communicates with you and bends her/his legs to place the feet on the mat.

3. Your partner will lower the chin towards the chest and use her/his core strength to stand.

4. Reverse roles and repeat the asana.

THE IDEA GUIDING THE ASANA

If you're the one below: This pose makes your hamstrings stretch.

If you're the one above: This asana works on your backward bend while also improving your sense of balance. You'll feel relaxed and taken care of, while also getting to observe the world from an unusual perspective.

AWARENESS

Your partner and you can focus on each breath and the connection between two bodies

If you're the one below: Observe how the alignment of your legs and your grip on your partner's wrists grant balance.

If you're the one above: Sense the touch of the partner's feet and hands on your body, and the kind of support this offers. Make yourself comfortable in a suspended stretch by relying on the trust you have in your partner and her/his ability to support you. Focus on letting go and look at the world as a hanging bat would—upside-down!

ASANA 32:
BEYOND THE BOW POSE

PREPARATORY ASANAS
Dhanurasana (asana 5)
Ustrasana (asana 7)

METHOD

Getting into the Asana

1. Lie down on your back, with your legs on the mat.
2. Let your partner stand, facing you, with her/his feet on either side of your ribcage.
3. When your partner starts to arch back, raise your legs to a 90-degree angle, keep the knees bent and feet flexed, and let your pointed toes touch the lower back of your partner.
4. Place both your hands firmly on your partner's knees.
5. Let your partner bend her/his knees till the body weight of your partner rests between your hands and toes.
6. Your partner bends her/his knees further so that the shins are parallel to the floor and off it.
7. Guide your partner such that s/he can hold her/his ankles and throw back her/his head.
8. Straighten your legs slowly while ensuring that your partner remains balanced on your feet.
9. Release your hands from your partner's knees and keep them by your side, the palms facing down.

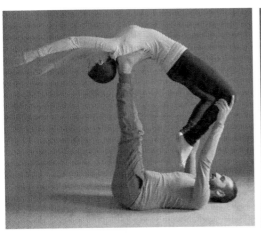
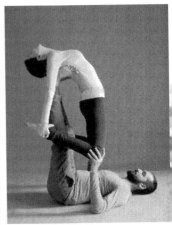

Maintaining the Asana

After following the sequence under 'getting into the asana', keep your hands firmly on the mat to maintain your balance, as also your partner's.

The partner above maintains a firm grip of her/his ankles. Your partner and you can breathe in and out, slowly and comfortably, holding the pose for about thirty seconds.

Coming out of the Asana

1. After following the sequence under 'getting into the asana' and 'maintaining the asana', your partner can release her/his right ankle and place the foot on the mat; s/he can then release the left ankle and bring that foot to the mat.
2. Once your partner's feet are down on the mat, you can push your feet into the back of your partner. Your partner comes out of the asana using the strength of the core and stands upright.
3. You may now lower your legs.

THE IDEA GUIDING THE ASANA

If you're the one below: This asana provides offers a unique stretch to the hamstrings and helps you settle the lower back on the mat.

If you're the one above: This asana allows you to practise a suspended ustrasana. In other words, you experience a backbend from a different perspective and get to deepen it further by exploiting the force of gravity.

AWARENESS

If you're the one below: Focus on your toes and observe how they are being pushed in while the heels are sliding out.

If you're the one above: Focus on the arch of the back as it deepens, especially making note of the impact of the force of gravity. Notice the support offered by the feet of your partner—they should grant you stability and comfort while you bend and balance. Also, remain conscious of the chest expanding with each inhalation.

ASANA 33:
TWO BRIDGES POSE

PREPARATORY ASANAS
Setu bandhasana (asana 6)
Ustrasana (asana 7)
Halasana (asana 20)

METHOD

Getting into the Asana

1. Your partner gets into sarvangasana (described as part of halasana in the 'getting into the asana' segment).
2. Slip into setu bandhasana, with your feet very close to your partner's shoulders.
3. Your partner slowly bends her/his knees and places her/his feet on your knees.
4. Your partner now releases her/his arms—thus far supporting her/his lower back—and stretches them until s/he can hold your hands. Ensure that you stretch your arms out, too, and clasp her/his hands.
5. Your partner will push the tummy forward so s/he can keep the back as straight as possible.

Maintaining the Asana

1. Both your partner and you can pull each other's arms towards one another.
2. Ensure that the position 'feels' tight and maintain it for about a minute.

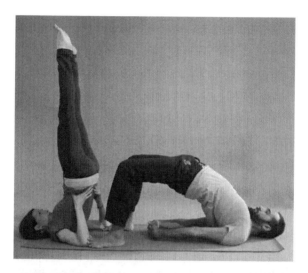

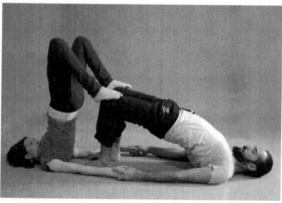

Coming out of the Asana

1. After following the sequence under 'getting into the asana' and 'maintaining the asana', release your partner's arms.

2. Your partner brings her/his hands to the back and supports her/his body. By keeping the legs totally straight and perpendicular to the mat, s/he can guide the body back into sarvangasana.

3. Both your partner and you will get out of sarvangasana and setu bandhasana (respectively), by following the sequence under each of these preparatory poses (under 'coming out of the asana').

4. Flip roles and repeat the asana.

THE IDEA GUIDING THE ASANA

In this asana, your partner and you need to work as a team to remain totally stable. This pose will also offer your thighs a stretch (along the front area).

AWARENESS

Your partner and you will focus on each intake of breath, and on the abdomen/chest going in and out while inhaling and exhaling. Both of you will also focus on the stretch offered to the front areas of the thighs.

You'll remain conscious of the dynamics of the pose. Observe how in this posture two bodies hold each other together. You'll feel a connection even if neither of you can see the other. Pay attention to the point of contact with your partner's body, and the support each gets via touch.

ASANA 34:
BRIDGE AND PLOUGH POSE

PREPARATORY ASANAS
Dhanurasana (asana 5)
Setu bandhasana (asana 6)
Halasana (asana 20)
Janu sirsasana (asana 22)

METHOD

Getting into the Asana

1. Your partner gets into sarvangasana (described as part of halasana in the 'getting into the asana' segment) and lowers her/his legs down, so s/he has now assumed halasana.
2. Lie down on the mat with your head pointing in a direction opposite to that of your partner's. Keep your feet close to her/his shoulders as you get into setu bandhasana.
3. While maintaining halasana, your partner now brings her/his arms down to the mat and reaches out for your wrists.
4. As you gently push your knees towards your buttocks, you pull your partner's arms towards yourself by the wrists.

Maintaining the Asana

1. After following the sequence under 'getting into the asana', you remain in setu bandhasana.
2. As you continue pulling your partner's wrists, s/he gets lifted by the tailbone, her/his toes slide away and s/he sinks further into halasana.

3. Your partner and you can hold the asana for about thirty seconds.

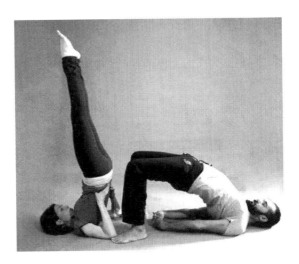

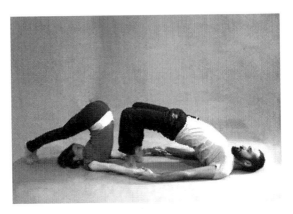

Coming out of the Asana

1. After following the sequence under 'getting into the asana' and 'maintaining the asana', your partner moves her/his knees

to the chest. This relieves some of the pressure and you can lower your hips back on the mat.
2. Release one another's hands, turn towards the side and arrange yourselves in any sitting position.
3. Flip roles and repeat the asana.

THE IDEA GUIDING THE ASANA

This asana acts as a counterposture to the previous one (asana 33 under 'partner yoga': the two bridges pose).

If you're the one in halasana: This partner yoga pose will help you increase the depth of your fold in a rather amusing way—after all, to maintain your balance, you need to reach out and grab the hands of your partner without seeing her/him.

If you're the one in setu bandhasana: You have to hold your partner's hands firmly, exerting just the right amount of pressure so s/he can maintain the pose with stability.

AWARENESS

If you're the one in halasana: Focus on the pattern of breath as you fold deeper into the asana. Make note of the support provided by your partner and the impact this has on your body.

If you're the one in setu bandhasana: Pay attention to those parts of your body in touch with your partner. Notice the impact that the pull of your hands has on your partner's capacity to fold her/his body.

ASANA 35:
BOW AND ARROW POSE

PREPARATORY ASANAS
Dhanurasana (asana 5)
Utkatasana (asana 8)
Shashankasana (asana 9)
Chaturanga dandasana (asana 17)

METHOD

Getting into the Asana

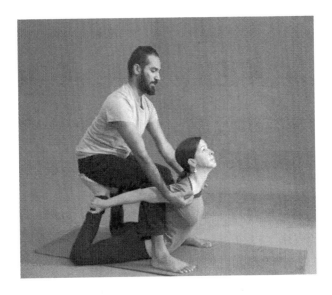

1. Your partner gets into dhanurasana and flexes her/his feet such that the soles face the ceiling.
2. Move into the space between your partner's arms, and align your shins with her/his torso.
3. Slowly bend your knees and lower your hips. Sit on the soles of your partner's feet.
4. Reach forward with your hands, hold your partner's shoulders and pull her/him back. This deepens the arch in your partner's lower back and allows her/him to expand the chest.

Maintaining the Asana

1. After following the sequence under 'getting into the asana', keep your spine straight and gently pull your shoulder blades inwards, to help your chest expand further.
2. Your partner deeply inhales into her/his expanded chest. S/he uses the back muscles to maintain a stable, well-balanced position for about thirty seconds while you sit on her/his feet.

Coming out of the Asana

1. After following the sequence under 'getting into the asana' and 'maintaining the asana', let go of your grip over your partner's shoulders.
2. Your partner now releases her/his ankles and lowers her/his hands down on the mat.
3. Reverse roles and repeat the asana.
4. Sink into shashankasana right after completing this sequence, since it acts as the ideal counterpose.

THE IDEA GUIDING THE ASANA

This asana is a lot of fun as one partner is literally sitting on the other's feet—as though on a chair.

If you're the one above: This asana helps strengthen your back muscles.

If you're the one below: This asana helps expand your chest. Moreover, since you have to shift your body weight towards your legs when your partner sits on your feet, you get to arch your body more emphatically than would be possible during an individual practice session of dhanurasana. The deepening of the arch grants a whole new set of impressions!

AWARENESS

Notice how two bodies support each other—with the body weight of one granting the posture steadiness, and the feet of the other acting as a stable chair!

If you're the one above: Remain conscious of how you maintain your balance on your partner's feet. As you gradually pull your partner's shoulders back, pay attention to her/his comfort levels.

If you're the one below: Inhale deeply and enjoy a supported backbend as well as the massage that is offered between the shoulder blades (which get squeezed towards the spine when your own arms and the hands of your partner pull your upper body back). Draw your attention towards the firm grip of your partner's hands on your shoulders.

ASANA 36:
GENTLE ARCH POSE

PREPARATORY ASANAS
Ustrasana (asana 7)
Shashankasana (asana 9)
Bhujangasana (asana 10)
Natarajasana (asana 18)

METHOD

Getting into the Asana

1. Lie down on your stomach with your arms near either side of your body.
2. Your partner stands facing you, with her/his feet on either side of your thighs/hips.
3. Your partner bends forward and holds your hands.
4. After communicating with you, your partner pulls your arms and lifts your chest off the mat by using the strength of her/his lower back muscles.
5. Your partner gently arches her/his back and lowers the head backwards.

Maintaining the Asana

1. After following the sequence under 'getting into the asana', continue to breathe normally.
2. Your partner keeps her/his eyes open and holds the pose for about thirty seconds.

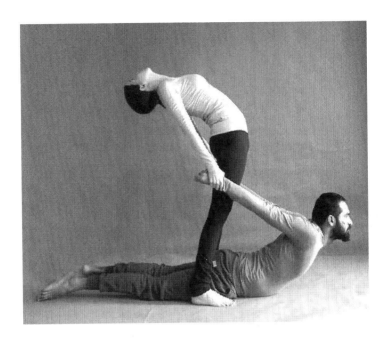

Coming out of the Asana

1. After following the sequence under 'getting into the asana' and 'maintaining the asana', communicate with your partner. S/he can lower the chin and pull back her/his hips to reduce the arch of the lower back and stand upright.
2. Your partner gently lowers your hands.

THE IDEA GUIDING THE ASANA

This asana—which makes both practitioners enjoy a supported backbend—is an effective but tricky counterbalancing pose.

It helps develop several life-skills—among them, good communication (so your partner and you remain stable and comfortable); trust (which is a necessary ingredient to complete the asana, since your partner and you don't face one another and cannot use sight to measure positions and reactions); and teamwork.

AWARENESS

If you're the one lying down: Learn to let go and trust your partner to attend to your backbend. Focus on your breath, the way it flows into your body, and how your chest and ribcage expand. Enjoy the massage offered between your shoulder blades.

If you're the one standing: Focus on the impact of your partner's body weight on your backbend, and make note of the influence this has on your balance. Don't miss the deep stretch offered to your back and arms.

Notice the kind of strength required to help your partner achieve a backbend, and ensure that you distribute your strength such that the weight of your body gets counterbalanced. Moreover, ensure that your partner's back isn't strained in any way, and avoid pulling her/him beyond her/his capacity to bear.

ASANA 37:
FLY WITH ME POSE

PREPARATORY ASANAS
Naukasana (asana 3)
Shashankasana (asana 9)
Kakasana (asana 28)

METHOD

Getting into the Asana

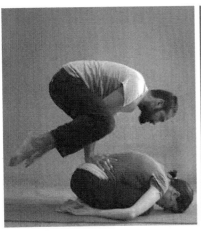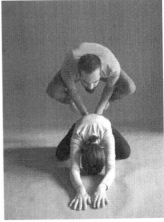

1. Your partner gets into shashankasana, with the knees wide, and lowers her/his chest between the knees.
2. Lace your hands and spreads your fingers wide on your partner's lower back.

3. Shift your body weight forward and balance yourself in kakasana on your partner's folded back.

Maintaining the Asana

1. After following the sequence under 'getting into the asana', use your core strength to hold this position and your arms to balance yourself while keeping your feet together.
2. Your partner breathes normally, relaxes her/his body and allows it to bend from the base of the spine. Your partner and you can try holding the asana for a few breaths.

Coming out of the Asana

1. After following the sequence under 'getting into the asana' and 'maintaining the asana', use your core strength to gently lower your feet to the mat and regain your balance. Stand up.
2. Your partner slowly comes out of shashankasana.
3. Reverse roles and repeat the pose.

THE IDEA GUIDING THE ASANA

This asana challenges your partner and you.

If you're the one above: This asana is extremely interesting since you have to balance yourself on the lower back of your partner.

If you're the one below: The pressure your partner applies on your lower back helps you slip even deeper into shashankasana. The body weight of your partner lowers your hips towards the mat, lengthens your spine and releases all tension from your lower back.

AWARENESS

If you're the one above: Make note of each breath and slow down your respiration. Focus on balancing yourself by activating the core muscles and extending each exhalation.

If you're the one below: Explore how it feels to provide support to the partner above. Make note of the pressure of your partner's hands on your back, and notice how your partner on top does not feel as heavy as you imagined her/him to be. On the contrary, your partner's presence is soothing, as your hips get lowered and your spine lengthens under her/his touch.

ASANA 38:
DOORWAY POSE

PREPARATORY ASANAS
Ustrasana (asana 7)
Shashankasana (asana 9)
Bhujangasana (asana 10)

METHOD

Getting into the Asana

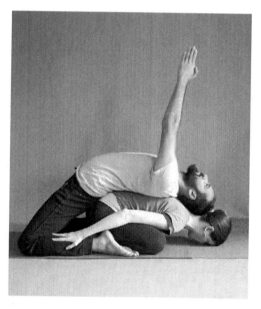

1. Your partner goes into shashankasana, bending forward.
2. Look away from your partner and get down on your knees.
3. Arrange your feet in such a way that the soles touch the thighs of your partner.
4. Raise your hands and arch back, your arms reaching for the ceiling.

Maintaining the Asana

1. After following the sequence under 'getting into the asana', relax the arch of your back on the curve of your partner's bent back.
2. Your partner keeps her/his knees as low as possible, and allows your weight to open her/his hips and fold still deeper into the position. Your partner and you can try holding this pose for thirty seconds.

Coming out of the Asana

1. After following the sequence under 'getting into the asana' and 'maintaining the asana', your partner places her/his elbows on the mat to keep the body from folding further.
2. Bring your arms back from over your head.
3. Your partner now presses her/his palms into the mat and keeps the arms straight. S/he slowly brings her/his body up, and with that, your body, too. Both of you are back to your starting positions.
4. Interchange roles and repeat the sequence.

THE IDEA GUIDING THE ASANA

If you're the one above: You receive the support you require to deepen the arch of your back; as you grow increasingly secure in the position, your chest expands and this improves the flow of breath.

If you're the one below: The weight of your partner helps you settle still deeper into shashankasana.

AWARENESS

Your partner and you focus on the point of contact between your bodies. You also focus on inhalations and exhalations, and the way each breath moves your bodies up and down.

If you're the one above: Notice how your body complements your partner's in this posture, and the soothing way in which your arch corresponds to your partner's deep fold.

If you're the one below: Observe the way in which the body weight of your partner is distributed. Also, don't miss the fact that while your partner's body helps you to fold deep into shashankasana, you enhance your partner's arch.

ASANA 39:
BUTTERFLY ARCH POSE

PREPARATORY ASANAS (TO BE PERFORMED
INDIVIDUALLY)
Padangusthasana (asana 2)
Baddha konasana (asana 4)
Ustrasana (asana 7)
Utkatasana (asana 8)
Natarajasana (asana 18)

METHOD

Getting into the Asana

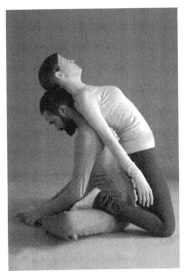
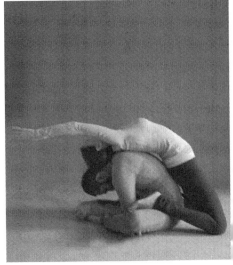

1. Get into baddha konasana and bend forward.
2. Your partner faces away from you and comes on her/his knees.
3. Your partner now arranges herself/himself such that her/his feet (from the top) touch your thighs.
4. S/he raises the arms and arches back, moving the arms over the head.
5. Your body folds.

Maintaining the Asana

1. After following the sequence under 'getting into the asana', keep your knees as low as possible and allow your weight to open your hips such that you fold even deeper.
2. Your partner relaxes the arch of her/his back on the curve of your bent back, and tries holding the pose for thirty seconds.

Coming out of the Asana

1. After following the sequence under 'getting into the asana' and 'maintaining the asana', place your elbows on the mat to prevent your body from folding further.
2. Your partner brings her/his arms back from over her/his head.
3. Now, press your palms into the mat and straighten your arms. This slowly brings your partner and you up, back to the starting position.
4. Interchange roles and start over.

THE IDEA GUIDING THE ASANA

If you're the one below: This pose improves your forward bend in baddha konasana, so the knees settle towards the mat.

If you're the one above: You get to comfortably arch your back and expand your chest, which promotes deep breathing.

AWARENESS

Your partner and you focus on the point of contact between your bodies. Besides, you also focus on every breath, and how inhalations and exhalations move your bodies up and down. Such attention to detail helps your partner and you experience the asana with greater intensity.

If you're the one below: Make note of the way in which the body weight of your partner is distributed. Focus on the soothing way in which your folding body corresponds to your partner's arched back.

If you're the one above: While your partner's body helps you deepen your arch, you help your partner fold her/his body better.

ASANA 40:
CARRY BAG POSE

PREPARATORY ASANAS
Naukasana (asana 3)
Dhanurasana (asana 5)
Utkatasana (asana 8)
Adho mukha svanasana or parvatasana (asana 12)
Garudasana (asana 13)
Matsyasana (asana 16)
Natarajasana (asana 18)

METHOD

Getting into the Asana

1. Your partner lies down on the mat and raises her/his arms, legs and chest using the lower back muscles. S/he takes the arms back and grabs her/his ankles by stretching the heels away from the hips, getting into dhanurasana.
2. Stand close, facing your partner, with your feet on either side of her/his waist.
3. Grab your partner from the ankles by bending your knees.
4. Keep holding your partner's ankles firmly and slowly start straightening your legs—this further arches your partner's back.
5. Your partner and you communicate with each other. Once both of you are comfortable in the pose, keep your legs and back entirely straight and lift your partner off the mat.

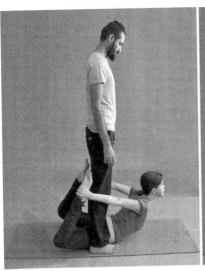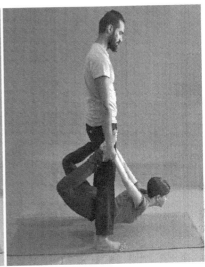

Maintaining the Asana

1. After following the sequence under 'getting into the asana', continue keeping your legs and back totally straight.
2. Your partner maintains the deep arch of her/his back and tries holding the pose for thirty seconds.

Coming out of the Asana

1. After following the sequence under 'getting into the asana' and 'maintaining the asana', gently lower your partner down and let her/his tummy touch the mat.
2. Firmly place your hands on your partner's lower back and soothe it. Then help your partner assume shashakasana (which is an effective counterpose) and relax.
3. After communicating with your partner, place your palms on her/his lower back, and gently massage the muscles surrounding the spine.
4. Reverse roles and repeat the asana.

THE IDEA GUIDING THE ASANA

Let's begin with a word of warning: Do not practise this asana if you have back problems.

If you're the one carrying: In this asana, above and beyond helping your partner deepen her/his arch, you need to offer reassurance and comfort.

If you're the one being carried: This position requires a very flexible lower back and supple shoulders that are comfortable with motion. You need to be aware of the dynamics associated with dhanurasana, since this pose makes you further deepen the arch offered by the preparatory pose, stretch your shoulders and breathe deeply. Besides being entertaining, this position reinforces your trust in your partner, improves your capacity to let go and helps you reclaim the playful moods of childhood.

AWARENESS

If you're the one carrying: Notice the kind of strength and security you offer your partner with your touch

If you're the one being carried: Pay attention to the parts of your body your partner focuses on to lift you. Observe how the element of trust plays an important role in this asana, as you rely on the grip of your partner to maintain your arch and balance. Feel your limbs stretch on account of the pull of gravity. Pay attention to your breath and hold on to a sense of calm during the backbend.

ASANA 41:
CHILD AND CAMEL POSE

PREPARATORY ASANAS
Ustrasana (asana 7)
Shashankasana (asana 9)

METHOD

Getting into the Asana

1. Allow your partner to settle down on the mat in shashankasana.
2. Stand behind your partner, bend forward and lay your hands on your partner's lower back.
3. Lower your partner's hips towards the mat, applying gentle pressure on her/him with the palms of your hands.
4. Place your feet on either side of your partner's hips, slowly lower your body down and sit on the lowest part of your partner's spine.
5. Communicate with your partner to ensure s/he is comfortable in the position.
6. Place your hands on your partner's shoulders and help her/him gently arch the back.
7. Reach out to your partner's elbows and slide your hands under them. Your partner keeps her/his hand over the head and joins the palms, as though offering a namaste.
8. Slowly pull your partner's elbows up—this will automatically lift your partner's torso further up.
9. Let your partner open her/his elbows; help her/him maintain this pose by placing your own elbows close to your knees.

10. Pull your chest up and hold your spine straight so that you increase the stretch offered to your partner.

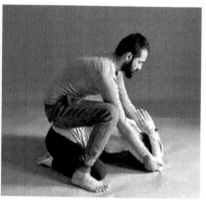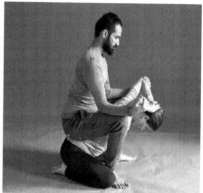

Maintaining the Asana

1. After following the sequence under 'getting into the asana', gently support your partner, urging her/him to close the elbows and bring them close to her/his face.
2. Tell your partner to stretch the arms up, and ask her/him to interlock the fingers around your neck.
3. Remind your partner to breathe in and out, slowly and deeply, while holding the pose for about thirty seconds.

Coming out of the Asana

1. After following the sequence under 'getting into the asana' and 'maintaining the asana', your partner releases her/his fingers from your neck. Guide her/his elbows, so they come together behind the neck in such a way that the palms convey a namaste, and the fingers point down.
2. Release your partner, stand up and let your partner rest in shashankasana.
3. Repeat the sequence, reversing roles.

THE IDEA GUIDING THE ASANA

If you're the one above: This asana allows you to deepen the arch of the partner below by bending *that* point in her/his spine which generally does not get arched during individual practice. It also helps you remind your partner to make the most of every inhalation, as her/his chest expands.

If you're the one below: In this pose, you can sense your chest opening and your triceps get stretched.

AWARENESS

If you're the one on top: Remain conscious of your partner's breath. Make sure that your partner is comfortable throughout the stretch by communicating with her/him at every stage of the asana.

If you're the one below: Sense the weight of your partner's body on your lower back and the beneficial impact of such pressure. Remain conscious of the stretch offered to your spine and the triceps; feel your chest open out. Note the soothing sensations in your spine and neck while you rest in shashankasana.

ASANA 42:
STORED PLOUGH POSE

PREPARATORY ASANAS (TO BE PERFORMED
INDIVIDUALLY)
Ustrasana (asana 7)
Halasana (asana 20)

METHOD

Getting into the Asana

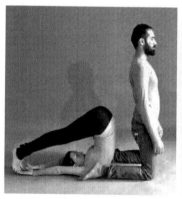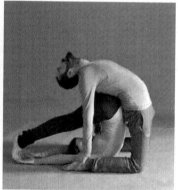

1. Your partner lies on the mat and gets into sarvangasana
    (described as part of halasana in the 'getting into the asana'
    segment).
2. Your partner brings both her/his legs down over the head
    and now gets into halasana, grabbing her/his toes.

3. Sit down on your knees, looking away from your partner, with your back close to her/him.

4. Lean back by arching your lower back—getting into ustrasana—using your partner's hips for support. Grab your ankles.

Maintaining the Asana

1. After following the sequence under 'getting into the asana', your partner (who is in halasana) keeps the hips lifted up. Resisting the weight of your arched body, s/he shifts her/his own body weight towards the shoulders by breathing normally.

2. After settling into ustrasana, rest on the arch on the buttocks of your partner, to get the support you need to further deepen the arch of your back; keep the head relaxed.

3. While your partner focuses on every exhalation, you focus on each intake of breath for about thirty seconds.

Coming out of the Asana

1. After following the sequence under 'getting into the asana' and 'maintaining the asana', come out of ustrasana by lifting one arm at a time. Sit on your knees, then stand up and move away.

2. Your partner releases her/his toes and uses her/his core muscles to regain balance.

3. Your partner brings her/his body back into sarvangasana and gently rolls out of the posture, vertebra by vertebra, till she is seated comfortably on the mat.

THE IDEA GUIDING THE ASANA

This asana offers support to your partner and you. While one of you will receive the bolstering you need to sink deeper into an arch, the other will receive the push required to melt into halasana.

AWARENESS

Experience the mutual support your partner and you give each other while performing this asana.

If you're the one above: As you bend back, focus on each intake of breath and the expansion of your chest. Notice how your back gets massaged by the pressure exerted by your partner's hips. Also notice how your partner's buttocks serve as a cushion to support the arch of your back. Remain conscious of the fact that, thanks to your partner's support, you can let go and enjoy the posture.

If you're the one below: Sense the pressure exerted on your buttocks and the area around the hips by your partner's body. Focus on each exhalation, let go and sink deep into halasana by exploiting the weight of your partner.

ASANA 43:
HAMMOCK POSE

PREPARATORY ASANAS

Naukasana (asana 3)

Dhanurasana (asana 5)

Utkatasana (asana 8)

Garudasana (asana 13)

METHOD

Getting into the Asana

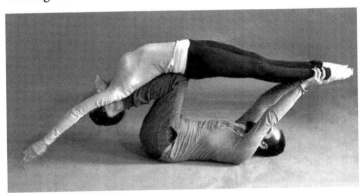

1. Lie down on your back on the mat.
2. Have your partner stand with her/his feet on either side of your hips, facing you.
3. Raise your legs such that they form a 90-degree angle with the floor.

4. Bend your knees and have your partner sit on them. Keep your legs firm and your thigh muscles, active.

5. At this stage, as your partner sits on your knees, her/his feet are still on the mat. Now, maintaining balance, your partner lifts her/his feet, one by one, as you hold her/his ankles.

6. Once your partner's ankles are firmly gripped in your hands, lift your feet up a bit and welcome your partner as s/he leans back on your shins.

7. Flex your feet and tuck the top of your feet into your partner's shoulders.

8. Your partner's legs stretch and remain straight, and your arms also become straight.

9. Your partner moves her/his arms over the head and relaxes. Her/his eyes remain open.

Maintaining the Asana

1. After following the sequence under 'getting into the asana', keep holding your partner's ankles.

2. Your partner stretches her/his entire body.

3. Your partner also keeps the back muscles relaxed to produce a uniform arch, and tries holding the pose for thirty seconds.

Coming out of the Asana

1. After following the sequence under 'getting into the asana' and 'maintaining the asana', communicate with your partner. Now, lift your legs further up.

2. Your partner uses her/his core muscles to lift the torso up.

3. Once your partner is upright and has regained a sense of balance, release your partner's ankles one by one.

4. Your partner stands up, and so can you.

5. Reverse roles and repeat the asana.

THE IDEA GUIDING THE ASANA

This asana is ideal if your partner and you wish to improve your balancing skills. Besides, this pose improves coordination and the capacity for synchronized movements. It helps lengthen and stretch the body and the upper back in an unusual and a rather playful way.

AWARENESS

This asana reminds you of the importance of communicating with your partner; after all, it can get a bit tricky! The partner above needs to slide along the shins of the one below, while the partner below holds her/him by the ankles, until a perfect height that matches the practitioners' build and size is found. Notice how a centre of balance is recovered naturally, and how both your partner and you can breathe calmly and normally despite holding an unusual position.

If you're the one below: Focus on the points of contact between your partner's body and your own. Note how the strength and support you offer is counterbalanced by the graceful stretch and arch of your partner.

If you're the one above: Relish the support and balance provided by your partner who holds you up. Enjoy lengthening your whole body, while hanging arched, in mid-air.

ASANA 44:
CLOSING 'OM'

PREPARATORY ASANA
Savasana (asana 11)
Sukhasana (asana 14)

METHOD

Getting into the Asana

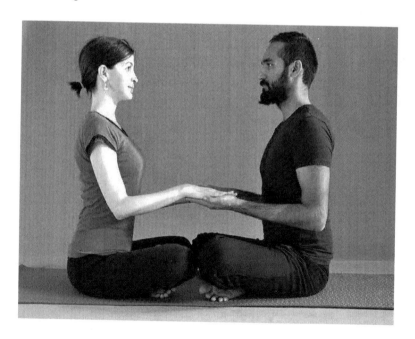

You are now ending your partner yoga session—and what better conclusion than the chant of a universal sound, 'Om'? Repeat this thrice, just as you did when you started the session.

Gently move out of savasana, which helped you relax at the end of your last posture. Keep your eyes closed, and without disturbing your partner's body, sit down on the mat comfortably.

1. Your partner and you sit in sukhasana, keeping the spine upright, and face each other.
2. Ensure that your knees touch your partner's.
3. Your partner and you will keep the right palm facing the ceiling and the left palm facing down.
4. Your partner places her/his hands on yours, so that both palms touch each other.
5. Both of you begin breathing slowly, attending to your own respiration, as also your partner's.
6. Take a long, deep breath together and start chanting 'Om', soaking in the power of the sound and keeping it at a stable frequency.
7. Chant 'Om' thrice.
8. At the end of the third 'Om', each partner rubs her/his palms, covers the eyes and then slowly opens them.
9. As you open your eyes, look at your partner with a welcoming smile.

THE IDEA GUIDING THE ASANA

The concluding chant helps your partner and you end the session harmoniously and peacefully. The syllable 'Om'—and the fact that you to attempt matching your partner's frequency—helps both of you acknowledge each other's presence. The position of the hands is a symbolic acknowledgement of the importance of giving and receiving.

AWARENESS

This concluding asana helps you exploit the many benefits of a partner yoga session—trust-building, focus, coordination and humility. As your partner's hands touch yours, you'll sense for yourself that this posture is unlike the opening one in the partner yoga sequence; delight in the ease and comfort you now have in each other's presence.

Tune into the vibrations around the spine produced by the sound of 'Om'. As you chant the mantra with your partner, notice how your breath keeps pace. When you open your eyes, do not forget to smile at your partner and thank her/him for sharing this session with you.

◆

If there is one life-lesson partner yoga wishes to gift all its practitioners, it is generosity—of giving unconditionally, and of receiving with joy. Hafiz sums it up, when he says:

> *Even after all this time,*
> *The sun never says to the earth,*
> *'You owe me.'*
> *Look what happens with*
> *A love like that.*
> *It lights the whole sky.*[1]

---

[1] Hafiz, 'The Sun Never Says', *The Gift*, translated by Daniel Ladisky (London: Penguin, 1999), p. 34.

ACKNOWLEDGEMENTS

Each time I have written the word 'partner' in this book, knowingly or otherwise, at the back of my mind, I have pictured my other half, Sara Atré. I want to thank her for staying awake night after night with me while revising the book, and accompanying me to Berlin, Amsterdam, London, Venice, Singapore, Thimpu, Manila and Delhi to help me find 'inspiration' and a suitable 'ambience' to complete the manuscript. I owe her a special thanks for making all this possible. You are the best!

I am deeply grateful to my parents, Manisha and Anil Atré, for believing in me and for their enthusiasm for my first book. I can't wait for them to hold this in their hands.

A big thanks to Sheekha and Ashish Atré for their love and support, and to Myer Ivan and Amayra for their daily dose of cuteness.

I am indebted to Isheeta Sumra, a very dedicated student and a dear friend, whose refreshing ideas have helped shape the book. You're awesome, girl!

A sincere thanks to my editor, Dharini Bhaskar, for encouraging me to write, keeping me focused during the drafting process and making my thoughts take the shape of words on pages. A high five!

Jumbo love to all my students who continue being my source of inspiration. See you all on the yoga mat.

Made in the USA
San Bernardino, CA
20 May 2017